workin' GIRL

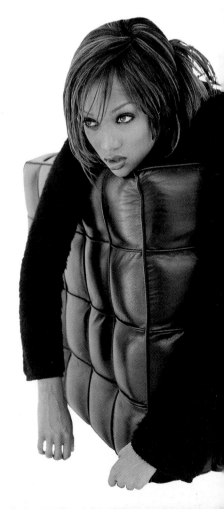

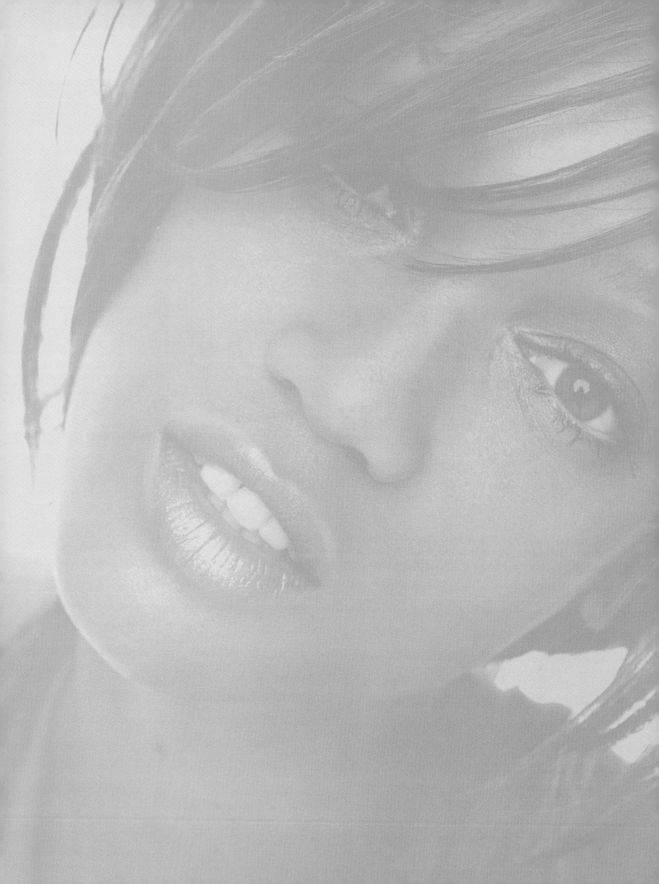

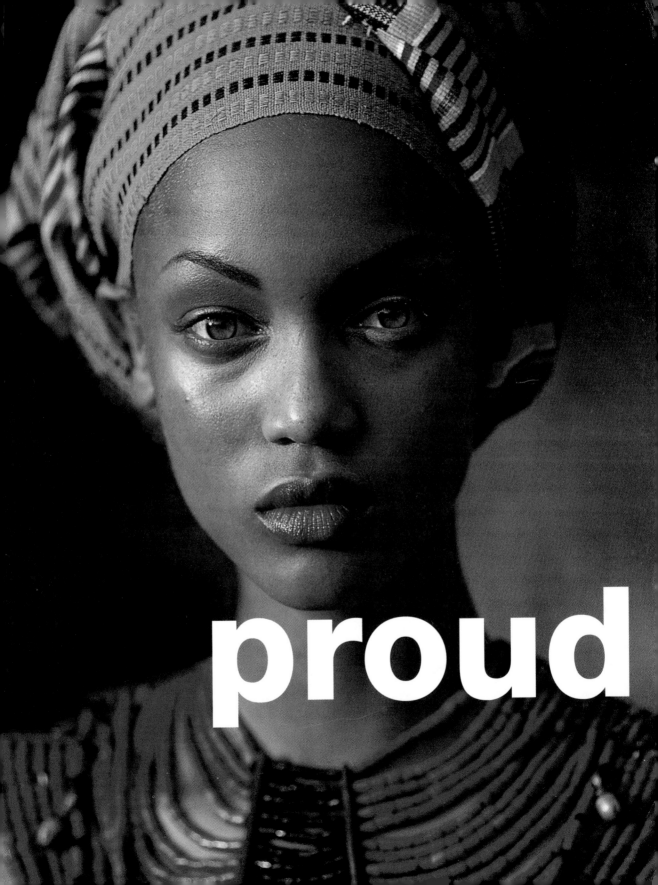

proud

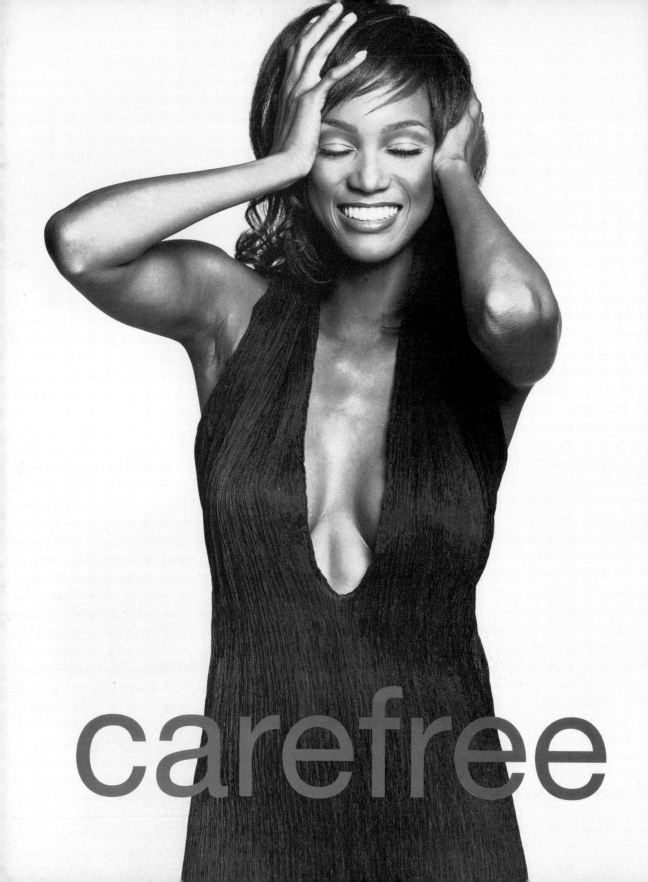

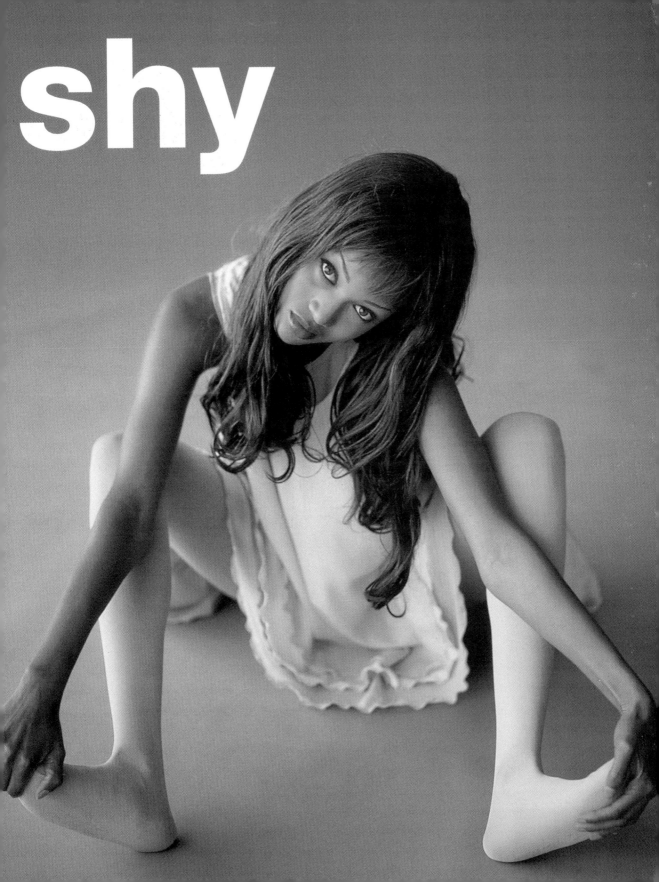

shy

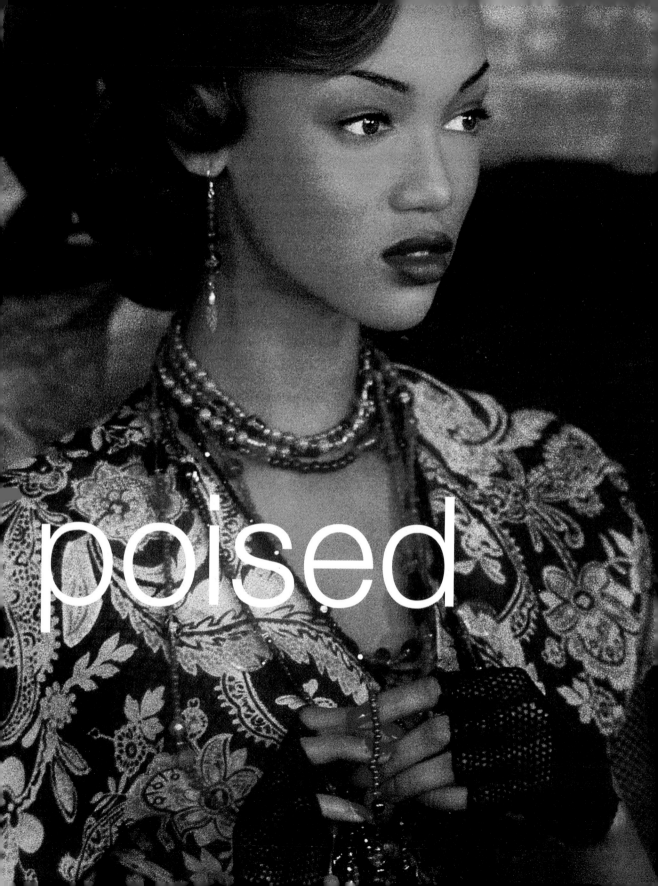

poised

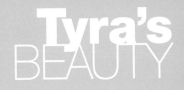

Tyra's BEAUTY

Inside & OUT

by
Tyra Banks

with
Vanessa Thomas Bush

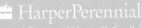
HarperPerennial
A Division of HarperCollinsPublishers

Acknowledgments

I want to give a big shout out to all of these amazing folks that made this book (which has been one of the most difficult things I've ever done in my life) possible.

HarperCollins
Kristen Auclair
Beth Bortz
Joseph Montebello
Susan Weinberg
Rose Carrano
Kristen Green

IMG
Chuck Bennett
Mia LoLordo
Jan Planit
Mark Reiter
Elaine Dugas
Maja Edmonston
Lisa Reiter
Jamie O'Conner
Vana Thayu

Service Station Design
Bill Anton
Dennis Favello

Photographers
Matthew Jordan Smith/
  Lewis Van Arnam
Gilles Bensimon
Carolyn London
Greg Henry
Mike Ruiz/Visages
Jonathan Mannion
Daniela Federici
Richard Hume
Betty Kitamura Fujikawa
Albert Sanchez
Tibault Jeanson
Sheila Metzner
Diane Franz
Andrew Dunn
Jonathon Glynn-Smith
Marianne Atkinson
Marc Baptiste
Bill Pollard
Moshen Saeedy,
  CM Color Laboratory

Gili Chen
Peggy Sirota
Annie Liebovitz
Troy House
Paolo Roversi
Walter Looss, Jr.
V.J. Lovero
Russell James
Bruno Bisang
Eli Reed
Kate Garner
Davis Factor
Hannes Schmid
Michael O'Neal
Kenji Toma
Antoine Verglas
Marc Hispard
Robert Erdman
Patrik Anderson
Dewey Nicks
Enrique Badulescu
Steve Granitz/Retna
John Spellman/Retna
Bill Davila/Retna
Jimmie Wilson, *photo assistant*
Briscoe Savey Jr.,
  photo assistant
Chris Spridigliozzi,
  photo assistant
Stephen Reel, *photo assistant*
Erskine Childers,
  photo assistant
James Kay, *photo assistant*

Special Thanks
Carolyn London
Don Banks
Devin Banks
Sharon London Burton
Bernetta Washington
Arielle & Tatiana Burton
Milan Bond
Marie Banks
Darilyn Banks
Demetrius Banks
Lindsey Rodriguez
Clifford Johnson, Jr.
Dominique Lebron
Amber Banks
Midnight
Keyser
Cindy Crawford
Tisa Gardner
Lisa Luke
Andrew Fox, *Esq.*

Mark Stankevich, *Esq.*
Carl Large, *CPA*
Marty Fox, *CPA, Bernstein,
  Fox, Whitman & Company*
Claudia Kowalchuk,
  *Bernstein, Fox, Whitman &
  Company*
Brad Cafarelli/
  Bragman Nyman Cafarelli
Lewis Kay/
  Bragman Nyman Cafarelli
Debra Jackson, *my amazing
  personal assistant*
Oscar James/Ken Barboza
Johnny Gentry/Ken Barboza
Tre Underwood
Sam Fine/Jean Owen
Troy Jensen/Celestine
Fran Cooper/
  LK & R Management
Billy B/Streeters
Edward G. Razek aka:
  "MISTER RAZEK"
Clayton James
Reggie Stiles
Peter Klamka
Claudia Schiffer
Robyn Roth
Cassandra Butcher
Monique Harris
Khefri Riley
Charlotte Wagster
Veronica Chambers
Jessie Collins
Todd Williams
Ruth Anne Murray
Toni Laudermilk
Anne Pajaud
Oscar Reyes
Francine Champagne
Prudence Hall, M.D.
Nicholas Hayek
Covenant House,
  Cheryl Trinidad
Paul Ludick
Iman
Jacklyn Wells
Arian Prescod
Jacqueline Prescod
Beverly Brooks and the Staff
  of The Center for Children
  + Families
Tyler Hills, *Timberlake and
  Timberlake West Camps*
Victoria's Secret

Swatch Inc.
Cover Girl
Marina Maher Communications
Disney Enterprises, Inc.
Sharon Chatmon Miller, *stylist*
Jessica Paster, *stylist*
Jennifer Danzi,
  assistant wardrobe stylist
Craig Gangi, *hair stylist/
  Heller Artists*
Candice Neil, *model/Bordeaux
  Model Management*
Lola Jean, *model/Bordeaux
  Model Management*
Jennifer Cohen, *model/
  Bordeaux Model Management*
Tracey Baudy, *model/
  Bordeaux Model Management*
Contrelle, *model/Bordeaux
  Model Management*
Shawna Erickson, *model/
  Bordeaux Model Management*
Nicholas Demps, *model/
  United Model Management*
Stanley Cuevas, *model/Boss*
Ruben Garcia, *model/Boss*
Zak Danielson, *model/Boss*
Ryan McTavish, *model/DNA*
Billy Teeples, *model/DNA*
David Lassiter,
  model/Wilhemina
Elion Chin, *model/Wilhemina*
Rick Passarella,
  model/Wilhemina
Craig Marshall, *model/Gillaroos*
Summer, *model/Next*
Anesha, *model/Elite*
Yaniece Thomas,
  model/L.A. Models
Michal Efrom Cohen
Bryan Rasmussen
Art Gray
David Parkett,
  photo researcher
Jamie Simmons,
  photo research assistant
Van Cleef & Arpels
Innovative Artists
Lewis Van Arnam
Audra Alexxi-Jones/
  Lewis Van Arnam
Milk Advisory Council
Mackie Mann
And last but not least,
Li'l Penny

*To the women before me who **paved** the way*

*To Daddy who **paid** the way*

*And to Ma who **paced** the way*

contents>

For information address
HarperCollins*Publishers*, Inc.
10 East 53rd Street
New York, NY 10022.

HarperCollins books may be
purchased for educational,
business, or sales promotional
use. For Information please write:
Special Markets Department
HarperCollins Publishers, Inc.
10 East 53 Street
New York, NY 10022

First Edition

Design by Bill Anton,
Service Station Design to Inform
and Promote, Inc.

Cover photograph by
Matthew Jordan Smith

Separations by Professional
Graphics, Inc.

Printed in U.S.A. by Quebecor
Printing, Inc.

Library of Congress
Cataloging-in-Publication Data

Banks, Tyra.
  Tyra's beauty inside and out/
Tyra Banks with Vanessa
Thomas Bush. – 1st ed.
    p.   cm.
  ISBN 0-06-095210-5
  1. Beauty, Personal.
  2. Cosmetics. I. Bush,
  Vanessa Thomas.
II. Title.
RA778.B225   1998
646.7'042–dc21   97-35345
                CIP

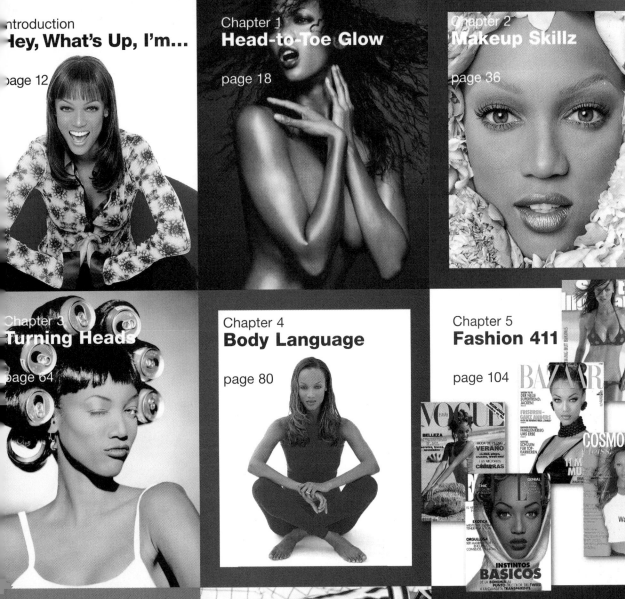

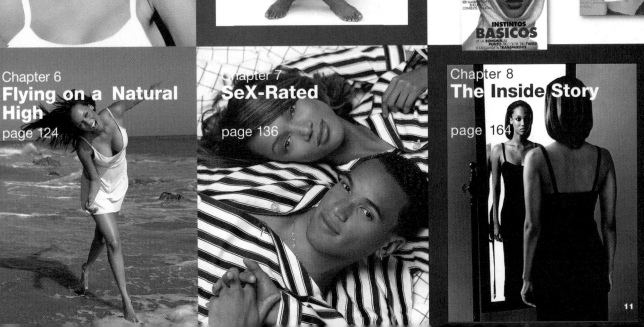

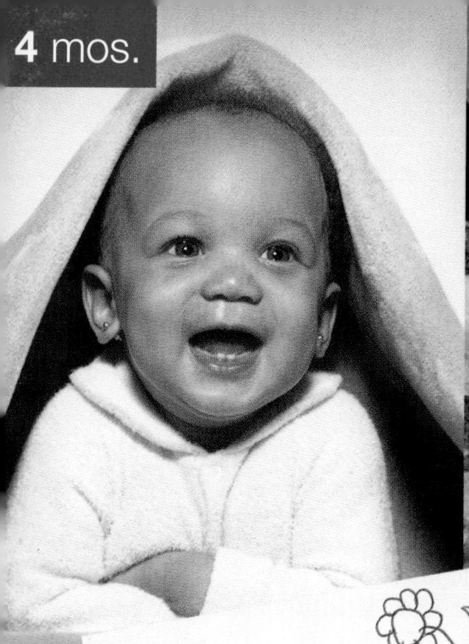

Giggling in my afro puffs

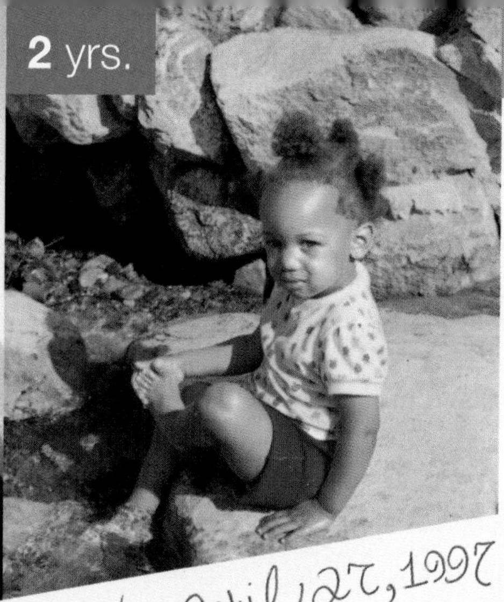

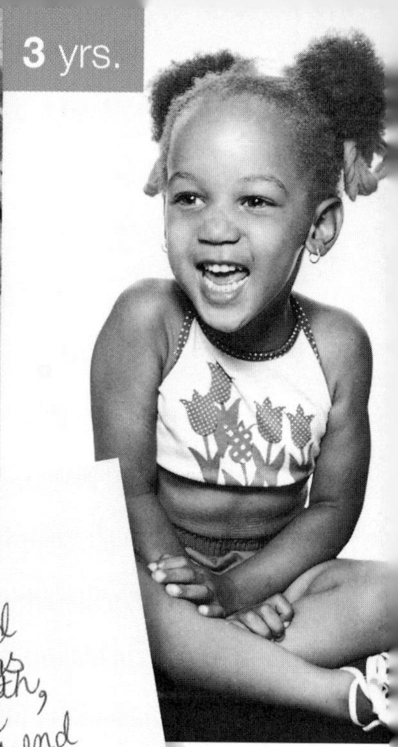

Introduction

April 27, 1997

Dear Tyra,
I am such a **HUGE** fan of yours. You are always so real and down to earth and you seem really happy. One of the things I admire most about you is your smooth, silky skin. I have tried every kind of makeup and skin cream but I only end up looking like a clown and breaking out in weird rashes and nasty 💥#%★*☹!

Me and my boyfriend have been having a lot of problems lately. Sometimes he sorta pushes me around and he slapped me (but only once). He says he needs a woman who respects him more. I'm so so so confused right now. I heard you say once that you don't have a boyfriend. Do you ever feel lonely or sad about not being with someone? I know I would!

I must sound like a big doofus asking you all these stupid questions. Maybe one day you'll visit my home-town and I can finally meet you in person. But who am I fooling? That will probably never happen.

Oh well, it doesn't hurt to dream...

Your #1 fan, Tracey Walker

12

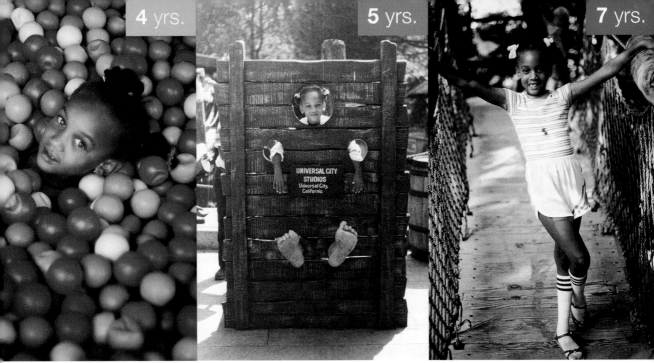

Stylin' & Profilin'

HEY
What's Up, I'm

Tyra Banks

Two years ago, when I decided to write a book on beauty and self-loving, I had several goals in mind. I get thousands of fan letters every year—with questions asking about makeup, hair, men, clothes, friends, and working out—and I wanted this book to be my "answer" to all of you. There are a million books out there that tell you how to apply lipstick, but I wanted to lay it **all** out on what really makes a woman beautiful, and I wanted to be open and honest on everything from sex and dating to substance abuse to self-empowerment. And, of course, I wanted to share the beauty and fitness tips I've picked up and perfected over the past six years by working with some of the finest experts on the planet.

So I got to work, pulling together all kinds of up-to-date information, browsing through old journals, flipping through my beginning modeling portfolios and photograph albums. It really took me back. (Don't laugh; I know some of the pictures are kinda funny-looking.) As I sat on the floor shuffling through all of these old photos, I couldn't help but ask myself, "How did I, Tyra Banks from Inglewood, California, become a supermodel?" It wasn't that long ago that I was a young girl dealing with the same insecurities, fears, and negative thinking that I read about in these girls' letters every day. (In fact, I'm *still* dealing with a lot of those same issues.)

They tell me that they cut out photos of me and plaster my image all over their walls. They say that they look at me as being "perfect" with not a problem in the world. If they could only see me on those days when I'm locked in the bathroom the night before a big photo shoot with a terrible

Think ya got the LOOK?

Keep workin' it, ya never know...

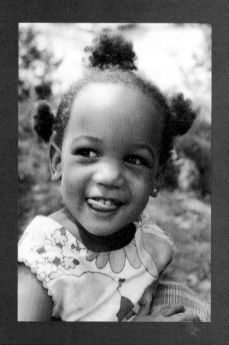

case of stomach cramps, or when I'm holed up in my room feeling down in the dumps and heartbroken over some big breakup.

People seem to have the idea that since I am in the public eye and often called a role model, I am above the normal human experiences of pain, self-doubt, rejection, and physical imperfections. I know I am successful in my job, yet I still do not see myself as this "famous celebrity" the way others do. As long as I've been in this business, I'm still amazed when I see a huge crowd of fans show up for an autograph signing, or when photographers jump in my face, clicking away, both at my public appearances and in my private life. Sometimes I turn around to see who they are waiting for, and when I realize that it's me, I have to laugh and shake my head.

With my success, I have seen drastic changes in how people treat me and react to me, but I've tried not to let all of this

ELLE

100 FASHION TREASURES

100 BEAUTY PLEASURES

ALL WE WANT FOR CHRISTMAS

THE ELLE 200

PARTY CLOTHES
SIX DEGREES OF BLACK TIE

SWEARING OFF SEX
THE YOUNG AND THE CHASTE

STEPHANIE SEYMOUR:
HOW A MODEL MAKES UP

ON THE SET OF "LITTLE WOMEN"

NUTRI-NONSENSE #171:
THE DEEPAK CHOPRA DIET

THE SWIMSUITS YOU'LL ACTUALLY WANT TO WEAR

DECEMBER 1994
USA $3.00
CANADA $3.50

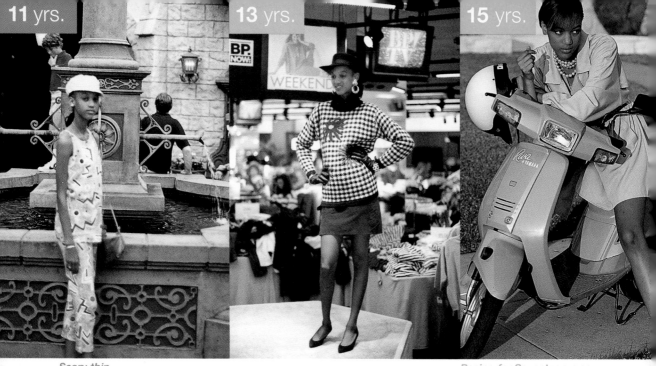

11 yrs.

Scary thin

13 yrs.

15 yrs.

Posing for Seventeen mag

"All I can do is try to tell my story openly and honestly."

special treatment affect my perspective. It's hard for some people to accept that I can be as good-natured and down-to-earth as I seem. Some think that it is all an act. When I was giving a lecture at Georgetown University last year, a young woman in the audience challenged me on my subject, which was self-esteem. With much attitude, she asked, "Why did you come here to speak to us about self-esteem when you have every reason to feel good about yourself? Not every woman can look like you do." I could have gone into the fact that modeling is just a job, or that everyone has some special talent they can be proud of, or a number of other things, but my answer was simply this: "All I can do is try to tell my story openly and honestly of what I have experienced." She seemed dissatisfied with that response; she sucked her teeth and sat down with a "whatever" expression on her face.

I hope she will read this book and understand me better. Still, there are those who will resent me no matter what I say and do. It's hard to deal with sometimes, but I now realize that I can only be myself and not let the negative energy of others get to me.

I know some people may still say they don't want to listen to someone whose life seems to be so full of glamour, where everything is handed to her on a silver platter. Well, if you think that, take a look at some of the photos above and on the previous pages. As you can see, I was not brought up by super-rich and famous parents, and I've actually had a pretty normal life.

SOON YOU WILL BE GETTING THE REGCOG... ...ON YOU DESERVE

FAME AND FORTUNE LIE AHEAD

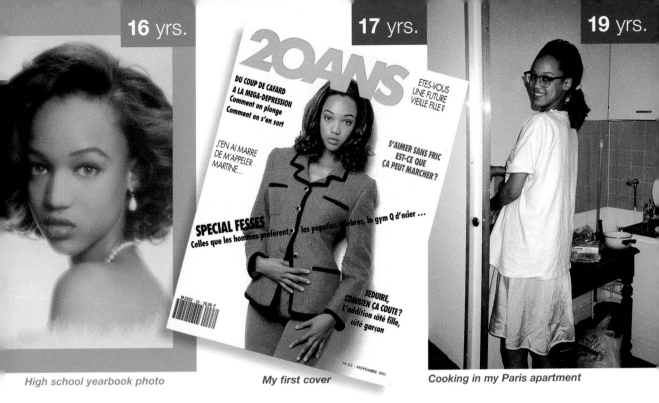

High school yearbook photo

My first cover

Cooking in my Paris apartment

I have genuinely had some troubling experiences, from agonizing over my super-thin body in adolescence to major problems with the opposite sex. I look back and laugh at how dramatically I dealt with some past issues—crying, screaming, wanting to run and hide, or just giving up altogether.

Yes, I do accept that I have achieved a great level of success in a career that makes a big deal about physical appearance. Fortunately, I was taught at an early age that physical beauty isn't all it's cracked up to be and that pretty faces come a dime a dozen. We are in our bodies for life, so we should make the most of them by taking a positive approach to how we look and feel. I've also learned that there are also more important things in life, like staying true to your beliefs, forming close friendships, developing an independent mind, being fit and healthy, and most of all, learning to love yourself.

What you have in your hands now is a compilation of many of my life's lessons. Although I have traveled the globe and have seen a lot, by no means am I an expert. In the pages that follow, I share my personal experiences. I like to collect interesting tidbits of information—my friends call me the "factoid queen"—and I've sprinkled many of these fun facts throughout the book. But when things get technical, you'll see that I turn to the knowledge of experts.

I hope as you read this book it will not only teach you neat tricks of the trade, but that it will also help you reach into the deepest spaces of yourself and encourage you to accomplish whatever you choose.

So are you ready? Well, here we **GO...**

1

Head-to-Toe

When I was growing up, I suffered from all kinds of skin ailments. The warts I developed when I was about nine years old were the worst of it. I had a chronic case of them on my fingers that was so bad the kids in my class called me "Froggy."

I walked around with gloves on in the summer, and wore clothes with pockets just to keep my hands out of sight.

I used to complain to my parents about the warts, but they assured me that I'd simply outgrow them. Well, those warts weren't going anywhere. After months of tears and whining, my dad took me to see a dermatologist. The doctor used some liquid nitrogen to freeze them and they eventually fell off. After a few treatments, they stopped appearing.

GLOW

Because of my chronic wart episode, I was a little self-conscious about my skin, but my aunt helped me overcome that. She convinced me that the warts weren't my fault, so I shouldn't waste time worrying about them. She encouraged me to expend that energy taking care of things I *did* have control over, like keeping my skin healthy and soft.

Aunt Sharon believes the body only gives as good as it gets, so she taught me that keeping the skin in good shape should be a natural extension of my health care routine.

I've always been thankful for that early guidance, especially now that I do so much swimwear and lingerie work. Those helpful hints really came in handy with my first *Sports Illustrated* swimsuit issue. I had to expose my face and body to some harmful elements—hot sun, burning sand, and frigid water temperatures. If I hadn't already learned to take certain precautions, I might have wound up with chapped, itchy, irritated skin, and there's nothing photogenic about that.

My years in the business have taught me that the camera doesn't lie. If I have a pimple, dark spot, or rough patch, it will definitely show up in a photograph. And while it's true that photographers do use retouching to erase noticeable blemishes, too much retouching can become expensive. That's why advertisers prefer to hire models with skin as flawless as possible. (Nice teeth aren't a bad asset either— but we'll talk about that a little bit later on.)

After years of fine-tuning, my regimen is so tried and true that I'm completely confident in what it can do. If you haven't found just the right routine, don't worry, because with a little bit of experimentation, you will eventually hit on one that works for you. After that, the secret to healthy skin is simple: **With the right products and regular maintenance, you'll always be ready for your close-up.**

the
body
only
gives
as
good
as it
gets

The Naked Truth

have desert-dry skin, so I concentrate on keeping it well moisturized. Exfoliaton and moisture-rich lotion are lifesavers for me. Depending on the state of your skin, you might need to take a different approach. If you're unsure about what skin type you have, here's a chart that might help:

SKIN TYPE	Characteristics
Dry	Dull, flaky complexion caused by underproductive oil glands. Skin absorbs moisturizer, and is still thirsty for more. Skin feels tight when you open your mouth wide.
Oily	Very shiny complexion, caused by overactive oil glands. Pores are often clogged, resulting in pimples.
Combination	The t-zone (across the forehead, down the nose, and chin) is oily; the eye and cheek areas are dry and sometimes flaky.
Normal	Skin is neither dry nor oily; it's just right (you lucky dog!). Complexion is smooth and problem-free.

Because face and body are not one in the same, you will need to treat them as separate entities. Most faces respond well to a routine that includes **cleansing, toning, and moisturizing.**

Cleansers remove the grit and grime our skin soaks up every day. I wash my face twice a day with a white washcloth so I can see how much dirt I'm removing. (I keep a large supply of white washcloths on hand for this purpose.)

Many people believe that if you don't wear makeup daily, you don't need to wash you face every day. But the pollution in the air is enough to clog anyone's pores. Our body's natural secretions—sweat and oil—also attract grime.

That's why toners are so important. They act as backup, clearing away whatever residue the cleanser doesn't catch. They also close pores and tighten and firm the skin, giving it a smoother appearance.

Because toners contain agents that could be drying, they should be followed up with a moisturizer. Moisturizers hydrate the skin with softeners that restore the skin's moisture balance. I prefer the kind that contain sunscreen because it gives my skin that extra layer of protection.

Keeping your skin clean can be costly, but it's not necessary to spend a lot on a fancy skin care system. Most of what you're paying for with those expensive products is the designer name and pretty packaging, but there are plenty of products in your local drug store that work just as well.

What matters more than price is how the product performs. Knowing your skin type narrows down the field. After that, it's all about experimenting. The key is to find a skin regimen that satisfies your concerns without creating new ones. Here's how to make sure a product is working for you and not against you:

Dry Skin	
Cleanser	Should soften and soothe the skin, leaving it supple, not dry.
Toner	Gentle, alcohol-free formulations that won't deplete the skin of moisture.
Moisturizer	Thick, rich creams that replenish and retain moisture work best.

Oily Skin	
Cleanser	One that is oil-free is an absolute must.
Toner	Versions that keep oil under control without overdrying.
Moisturizer	It should be oil-free, yet replenish moisture.

Combination Skin	
Cleanser	One product to keep the t-zone (forehead, nose, and chin) free of pore-clogging oils, and another to keep the eye, cheek, and neck areas cleansed without drying them out.*
Toner	An oil-free version for the t-zone; an alcohol-free version for the rest of the face and neck.*
Moisturizer	An emollient-rich product for the eye, cheek, and neck area; the t-zone may not require anything.

Normal Skin	
Cleanser	A mild product that isn't too drying or too oily.
Toner	Mild and alcohol-free.
Moisturizer	A light lotion to keep skin hydrated.

*Note: If you invest in a product line that is safe for all skin types, you can save a few dollars.

7:00-7:15 AM

Time to wake up, so I make a beeline to the bathroom. I grab my oatmeal cleansing bar and a white washcloth and start lathering up. I wash my face using a gentle touch so that I don't stretch out or irritate my skin. I wash my entire face, the front and back of my neck, then inside and behind my ears, being careful not to over-scrub because that can cause more dryness.

After rinsing with luke-warm water (hot water is too drying), I follow up with a toner. Some toners can be too harsh for my dry skin, so I dilute them. First, I soak a cotton ball with water, squeeze it out, then pour a little bit of toner onto the cotton. Then I sweep the cotton ball all over my face, avoiding my eye and lip area.

Next comes the most crucial step: moistur-izing. I make sure to cover everything, from my face and neck down to my collarbone. I don't wait until after I shower, because if I did, those areas would be overly dry and flaky. (I also take a few min-utes to brush my pearly whites, so that they'll stay that way.)

7:15-7:30 AM

I jump in a lukewarm shower, pull out a washcloth I use just on my body and start scrubbing. In the shower, I use a mois-ture-rich soap. I know some folks who like to mimic the commer-cials and just rub the soap all over their bodies. But that barely scratches the surface dirt. With a washcloth, I get rid of the grime and exfoliate in one step.

(About twice a week, I change up this routine a bit and use one of those scrunchy puffs or a loofah glove, instead of a washcloth, as an exfoliator. I don't use them every day, though, because they may slough off pro-tective layers of skin.)

Once I'm feeling fresh and clean, I step out of the shower and dry off a little bit, but I leave some dampness to work in with my lotion to trap in more moisture.

I like to use a thick, creamy lotion on my body, because it does not just slick up the surface, it sinks in. If I'm exposing my arms and legs, I use a lotion with sunscreen. And I never use the same lotion for my face that I use on my body—I tried it once in a pinch, and I broke out.

A lot of people only like to moisturize the areas that are exposed, but that's depriving your body of some valuable emollients. With me, the lotion goes on all over—arms, legs, breasts, stomach, butt, and back included. I also reapply moistur-izer to my face.

12:00 NOON

This is usually about the time when my face needs a boost, so if I'm not wearing makeup, I pull out a travel-size tube of moisturizer I keep in my bag and rehydrate my skin.

3:00 PM

I'm on an airplane heading to New York, and, as usual, the air on the plane is drying out my skin. I rarely fly with makeup on, so I pull out the spray bottle I've filled with water just for this pur-pose and give myself a couple of spritzes. I follow this up with some moisturizer. I do this every hour. If I don't, when I get off the plane my face feels like it's going to crack.

12:00-12:15 AM

I just got in from an event, and I feel like falling into bed right now, but I don't. I pull out the makeup re-mover. After wiping away the cosmetics, I repeat the face-cleans-ing and moisturizing routine from this morning. I also add a step—some petroleum jelly (or an inexpensive eye cream) around the eyes. I take a quick shower and moistur-ize my body all over again. Now I can go to sleep in peace, feeling totally relaxed.

Skin care really isn't all that time-consuming. It just takes a little commitment. When I stick to my routine, I rarely have any skin problems. When I don't, I wind up planted in front of the bathroom mirror, worrying about how I'm going to cover up my new pimples. All this can be avoided if we consistently give our skin the attention it deserves.

Bad News Breakouts

When I'm working, I can have up to five different sets of hands a week touching my face at the makeup table. They use all types of cosmetics with ingredients that may or may not agree with my skin and can cause breakouts.

For the most part, I've been lucky. My skin doesn't break out all that often. But when it does, it can be pretty nasty. I get huge, bright-red raised bumps with a head of white pus smack-dab in the middle that just begs to be popped. But I don't succumb to the temptation. I'm careful about the way I treat them so there won't be any reminders (like scars and dark spots) after the pimples are gone.

Thankfully, there are some surefire ways to combat these outbreaks:

Four Breakout Busters

1 Drink plenty of water–it flushes out impurities, ridding the body of toxic substances that can build up and cause skin problems.

2 Keep your hands away from your face to avoid spreading germs.

3 Wash makeup brushes and sponges frequently to minimize dirt and bacteria.

4 Pull hair back away from the face when possible. Bangs and similar styles can transfer hair oils onto the face and cause breakouts.

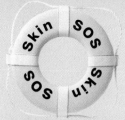

Whenever I can, I try to handle my skin problems on my own. But there are some that are too serious to tackle at home and that I think should be strictly a dermatologist's domain. If you are experiencing any of the symptoms below, don't try to handle the problem yourself. Instead, schedule an appointment with a professional.

Moderate to Severe Acne
The signs: Breakouts and, sometimes, facial scarring. Acne is caused by overactive oil glands due to hormonal changes, and the oil gets clogged in the pores and becomes infected.
Remedy: A dermatologist might recommend creams or lotions such as vitamin A acid or benzoyl peroxide, or might prescribe an antibiotic such as tetracycline, minocycline, or erythromycin to reduce redness and bacteria. She may also inject cortisone directly into the bumps or prescribe oral medications such as isotretinoin.

Eczema/Atopic Dermatitis
The signs: Reddened, brownish, scaly, itchy, irritated skin that sometimes looks like a rash. Anything from the fragrances in detergents to showers that are too hot can trigger a breakout. Sometimes it's simply heredity.
Remedy: A dermatologist might recommend cortisone ointments, tar creams, lotions, or oils to soothe the skin. Antihistamines may also be prescribed to control the itching. In severe cases, ultraviolet-light therapy might be used.

Hyperpigmentation
The signs: Dark spots caused by picking pimples, insect bites, or other trauma to the skin. The condition is more commonly found in women of color. There is little scientific evidence to prove that over-the-counter fade creams will erase the problem, despite the millions that consumers spend on them each year.
Remedy: A dermatologist might suggest an alpha-hydroxy acid or a prescription-strength fade cream that can help reduce the discoloration.

Viral Warts
The signs: These skin growths–sometimes raised, sometimes flat–are caused by a virus. They are contagious and can spread from one part of the body to another.
Remedy: Dermatologists can't kill the virus, but they can destroy the outer layer of skin where the wart grows. Removal methods include freezing the wart with liquid nitrogen or with chemicals like salicylic acid, laser ablation, or surgery.

Melanoma
The signs: Changes in the shape, surface, or color of a mole; a bump that bleeds or oozes; pigment of a mole that runs outside its normal borders and into the surrounding skin (edges are blurred or blotchy-looking). Excessive exposure to the sun is the primary cause.
Remedy: Doctors recommend periodic self-exams to learn the shape, color, and frequency of your own moles. If their appearance suddenly changes, or if a new mole appears that wasn't there before, you should immediately consult a dermatologist. If caught in its early stages, melanoma is curable.

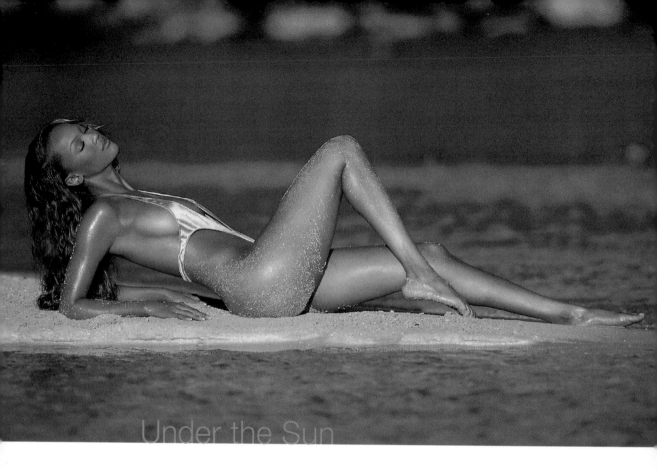

Under the Sun

There was a time when I used to expose myself to the sun without any protection—no sunscreen, no hat, no nothin'! I figured, "I'm black, so my skin won't burn." Unfortunately, I had bought into the myth that people with darker skin tones don't need sunscreen. I thought the melanin in my skin was enough to keep the sun's rays from doing any harm.

I learned my lesson the hard way, on a modeling job in the Caribbean on the island of Anguilla. We finished early in the day, and I had some time to chill, which to me meant grabbing a plastic raft and heading for the nearest beach. Well, I laid my non-sunscreen-wearing butt on that raft and floated along the shoreline until I fell asleep. When I woke up hours later, I had a golden tan that I was ecstatic about. But by the time I was ready for bed that night, my skin was hurting. I didn't understand why. I thought maybe I was allergic to my new skin lotion or the detergent the sheets were washed in. I couldn't get comfortable and every time I moved, my skin ached something terrible.

The next day, when I told the other models about my sleepless night, they knew immediately what the problem was, because they had been there many times before. *I was sunburned!* It had never occurred to me that that was the problem. Soon enough, it became painfully obvious, because I started to peel. First my chest started to blister, then dry, damaged layers of skin started shedding off me in sheets. I was a mess!

Ever since then I have worn some kind of sun protection, typically a sunscreen with an SPF of fifteen. I use one type for my body and a gentler one for my face. And I try to wear a hat with a wide brim as often as I can.

An SPF of fifteen isn't like a total eclipse of the sun—some rays will still get through, just not with the same intensity as they would if you went without any protection.

When skin burns, it's serious business. The epidermis (outermost layer of skin) is our only protection against the elements. If that protective layer is damaged, it leaves us open to all types of health concerns, including skin cancer. No tan is worth all that.

The easiest way to make sure you're well covered is to put on some sunscreen before you ever set foot outside. Sun protection isn't just for the beach—the sun's penetrating rays are just as damaging whether you're doing some window-shopping or working in the yard. I use sunscreen daily, and when I'm wearing makeup I layer it on underneath. (Some cosmetics companies even offer makeup with protective ingredients.) If I'm doing something where I'm really active, I use a sports sunscreen because it's less likely to wear off when I'm working up a sweat.

Sunglasses and a hat are protective measures that add another line of defense against sun damage. Clothing that covers most of your body is another barrier. Instead of catching rays, make catching some shade your main priority; your skin will thank you.

Taking It *Off*

I love being a woman, but there are times—like when I have to go in for a bikini waxing—that I wish I were a man so I wouldn't have to deal with hair removal. It doesn't seem fair that they should be able to walk around all hairy and not care a bit, while most women are afraid to be seen on the beach in a bathing suit if that bikini line hasn't been waxed or shaved.

I refuse to obsess over hair removal. I only shave my armpits when I know I'm going to wear clothes, like a sleeveless shirt, that will expose the hair. The hair on my legs is a light color, and sparse, so I don't shave them at all, not even for photo shoots. I've never seen my leg hair show up in an ad, so until it does, that's one step I'm happy to skip. I also have a very fine, but noticeable, mustache on my upper lip that I tried waxing off, but found the pain unbearable. So I use a bleach that lightens the hair instead of removing it.

Hair removal is no picnic; in fact, sometimes it can be a pain! Between the razors, the waxing, the depilatory lotions, and (ouch!) electrolysis, it almost sounds like torture. (More power to the women who refuse to shave—you go, girls!)

I've tried almost every removal method, and here's what I think are some of the pros and cons. I've also rated each one's comfort level on a scale of one to ten, with ten being the most comfortable. Of course, how long each method will last is really a matter of your personal hair-growth pattern.

Shaving

Pluses	Minuses
Quick and inexpensive	Doesn't last long; stubble reappears quickly
Easy to do at home	Possibility of nicks and cuts if you shave too closely; could lead to infection

Comfort Factor: 8

The key is to drench the skin with water and use a moisture-rich shaving cream and a soothing lotion to soften the skin afterward.

Waxing

Pluses	Minuses
Removes hair close to the root; leaves skin smooth	Causes some pain and soreness
Can last for weeks	Costs more than shaving, whether done at home or professionallly

Comfort Factor: 4

Waxing can remove a layer of skin along with the hair. To minimize the pain and swelling, take an antihistamine about an hour before waxing. Follow-up with a soothing cream.

Depilatories

Pluses	Minuses
Easy to apply	Unpleasant odor
Inexpensive	Chemicals may cause skin to sting

Comfort Factor: 9

The risk of any stinging is mild, but to lower those chances, do a patch test on a small area before you use it on the entire section. To minimize irritation, try not to exfoliate beforehand. It's best to use a depilatory that comes with built-in skin soothers, then follow with a thorough rinsing and moisture-rich cream.

Electroysis

Pluses	Minuses
Stops hair growth forever because it deadens hair follicles	Should only be performed by a professional, which can be costly
	Have to go for repeat visits, because the first treatment doesn't always remove the hair permanently.

Comfort Factor: 1

Because you are sending electric current directly to the hair root, the pain can be intense. Taking aspirin or ibuprofen before the procedure has been known to help. An operator can also apply a topical anesthetic to numb the area beforehand.

Should You
Tattoo?

Five years ago, tattoos were such a big craze in the modeling world that you couldn't get undressed backstage at a fashion show without seeing one. Models were getting inked everywhere from their hands and legs to their stomachs and backsides. I toyed with the idea of getting one on my ankle, but I couldn't decide on a design that I could live with forever. In recent years I've reconsidered, but decided against it. I guess I'm just too chicken.

Aside from the fact that it's permanent, your biggest concern with getting a tattoo should be safety. I think that allowing a potentially harmful object to penetrate your skin means you should take a few precautions.

SEEK OUT EXPERTS.

Look for tattoo artists with experience; their expertise and professionalism is worth the expense.

CLEANLINESS IS KEY.

There is a risk of contracting hepatitis, HIV, and other infections from unsterilized instruments. Autoclaving–sterilizing the tools at 270 degrees before use–is the safest bet against problems.

THINK ABOUT IT.

Getting a tattoo is not a decision to make lightly. They are permanent, and if you want them removed, the process can be expensive, time-consuming, and painful.

CONSIDER THE ALTERNATIVES.

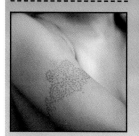

Henna tattoos (a.k.a. mehndi) are an attractive substitute for ink tattoos because they are temporary and painless. I've gotten an intricate henna design on my upper arm that was absolutely beautiful. The designs are made from a paste of finely ground henna leaves, which is left to dry on the body for from two to twelve hours. Henna tattoos last between one and two weeks (depending on how often you wash the tattooed area) and are done mostly on the hands and feet.

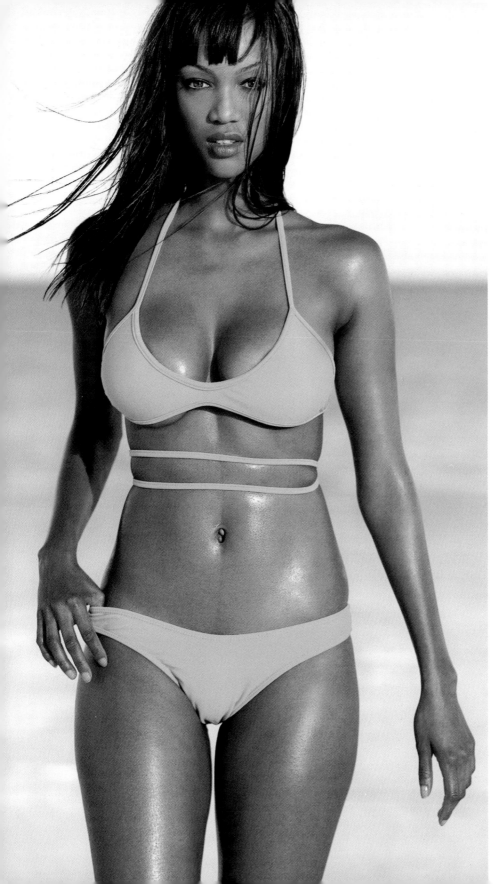

Pierced
Parts

I had my ears pierced when I was two months old, and to this day, those are the only piercings on my body. I wore a fake nose-hoop ring when I was seventeen, but I was never tempted to make it real. Many others, though, have dived into the body piercing phenomenon head first, getting everything from eyebrows, tongues, and lips to belly buttons pierced. Some things to remember if you decide to take the plunge:

Have the piercing done by a professional.

I know people who had their ears pierced by numbing their earlobes with ice cubes and making the hole with a sewing needle, but I think that's risky business. Make sure that the person who's doing the piercing is sterilizing the tools (preferably in an autoclave).

Keep an eye on your ears and other pierced parts.

When you first have them pierced, it's important to keep the area clean and disinfected with a deodorant-free, antibacterial soap and Bactine (or other solutions with benzethonium chloride) to avoid infection. (Some piercers also suggest using essential oils, such as lavender and tea tree, that have been diluted or antibiotic ointments if the piercing shows signs of minor infection.) Turn the earrings, nose ring, etc. every day to keep the hole from closing up.

great**whites**

The first time I went to the dentist I was six years old and I had eight cavities. I remember Dr. Smith, a mean and rough dentist who specialized in children's care but didn't seem to care about children. She jerked my head around and drilled my eight rotten teeth but wouldn't listen to me or give

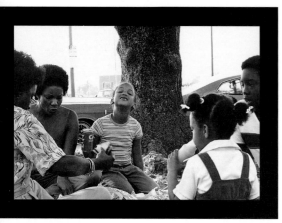

Showing off my snaggle-tooth grin

me more Novocain when I told her that I was in serious pain. When my mom found out how I was being treated, Dr. Smith was history. Her office is three blocks from my dad's house, and every time I pass it, I cringe.

I can see why so many people are afraid of the dentist. The sound of the drill alone is enough to keep anyone away. Many people have experienced what I have, or worse. For a lot of folks, just hearing other people's horror stories has kept them out of the dental chair.

But luckily, with today's technological advances, those fears are put to rest. Dentists now use methods of care that make most procedures pretty painless. There are topical anesthetics that dentists apply to the gums with a swab before a shot to temporarily numb the area; to help you relax, there are also antianxiety agents such as nitrous oxide that can be

inhaled. Some dentists even take a holistic approach by using aromatherapy and piping soothing music into the room to make you feel more mellow.

A beautiful smile is truly one of our greatest natural resources. With one upturned grin, our face lights up and lets our inner light shine! That's why dental visits should take place at least twice a year. In between, regular brushing and flossing are what it takes to keep teeth healthy and prevent gum disease. Here are a few pointers to keep those pearly whites sparkling:

a. Use a soft- or medium-bristle toothbrush; unlike hard ones, they won't irritate the gums.

b. Brush the tongue (especially in the back where food and bacteria can linger) to remove any residue.

c. Follow up with floss to remove food particles and plaque between the teeth. (The flavored kind keeps me from getting bored.) Sometimes I get lazy and don't floss, and my dentist can always tell. When I know I have a visit scheduled, I try to clean up my act and floss for two weeks before the appointment, but he says the only person I'm fooling is myself, and that if I don't want to wear dentures when I'm older, I better get to flossing regularly!

d. Finish it off with mouthwash and, voilà, a winning smile!

It's important to **brush a minimum of twice a day,** but it's best to do it after every meal. (I carry a travel toothbrush and toothpaste in my purse.)

A beautiful smile is truly one of our greatest natural resources.

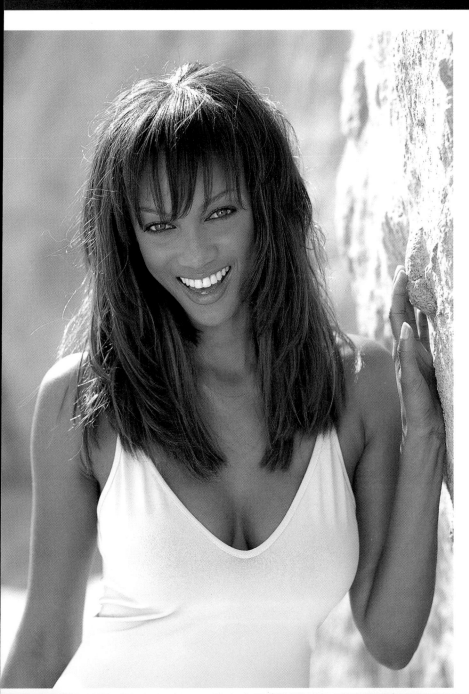

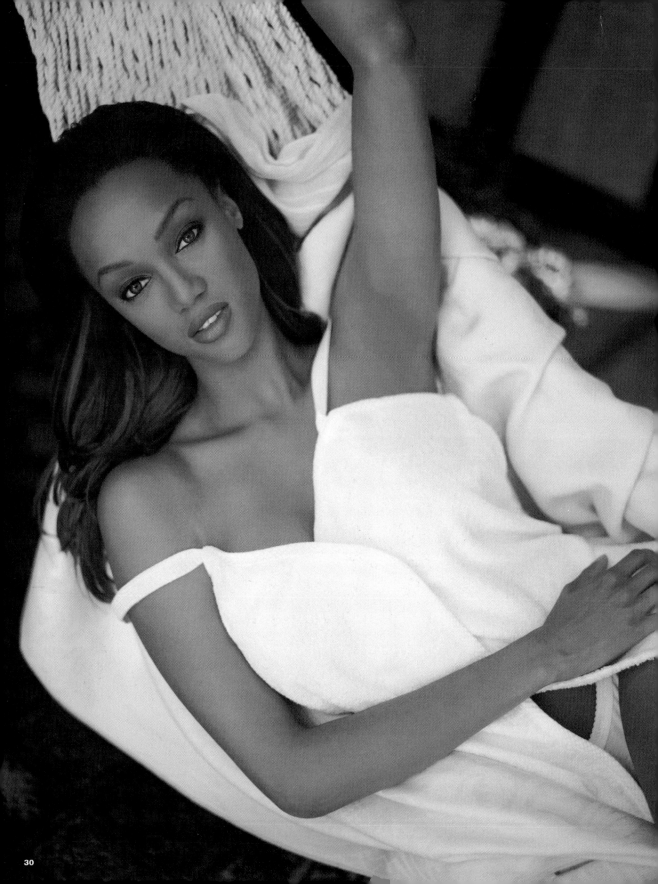

don't pamper myself the way I know I should. Like many people, I work a lot and the time I actually have to myself is minimal. When I do have a moment to unwind, the most I have energy for is a long, hot shower and a shampoo. Then I slip on my terry cloth robe and lounge around with some deep conditioner in my hair, a book on my stomach, and the remote to the TV within arm's reach.

On those rare occasions when I do treat myself to a spa visit, it doesn't take long to realize what I've been missing. There's a place in Los Angeles that's my favorite getaway. To me, it's an oasis. I love to take a soak in the hot springs (it's sort of like sitting in a hot tub, only the water is heated by nature), then cool off in the pool. I can just go back and forth like that for hours—the longer I stay in the water, the more relaxed I feel. The interesting part is that you see all kinds of body types there—round, slim, tall, short—but you don't have to worry about how you look because no one's self-conscious about it. I guess everybody's too busy kickin' back to care about what other people think.

After that's done, there's a communal room where you can go for a complete body scrub. First the spa ladies use a loofah on your entire body to scrub away dead skin cells and stimulate your circulation while they massage you. Then they put fresh, crushed cucumbers all over your body. Next, they pour honey and sesame oil all over you, on top of the cucumbers. Last, they bathe you from head to toe in fresh milk. I know, it sounds pretty sticky, but each step helps to refresh and renew the skin, and it's actually very soothing. When they're done, they wash everything off and then wash your hair, so you leave feeling squeaky-clean and completely spoiled.

When I really want to indulge myself, I follow the body treatment with a manicure and a pedicure. My hands are probably the most neglected part of my body. My aunt Sharon can attest to this. She can identify me in photographs by my wrinkly, rough, crooked-looking hands, even when my face isn't in the picture. And she's not the only one who notices. I get mail all the time from people telling me, "Tyra, you need to do something with your nails!" I got a French manicure once for the Victoria's Secret catalog and, judging by the amount of positive mail I received, those nails were a huge hit. It surprised me that people paid that much attention. It also told me that maybe a little hand pampering should become a regular part of my regimen.

The only problem with spoiling yourself at a spa is that it can add up, and quickly, anywhere from $50 to $1,500 or more. So I did a little investigating, and it turns out that some of the same beauty treatments they offer in the spas can be done **at home for considerably less.** All it takes is some beauty supplies and a few quiet hours all to yourself. I've pulled together a few at-home treatments, using products available at your local drugstore, that will give you the taste of an upscale spa without the hefty price tag.

scrub

TOOLS
Bath Oil (Baby oil does just fine.)
Mineral salts, available at your local drugstore
Scented lotion or cream
2 towels
Some candles and relaxing music (optional)

1

Run a bathtub with warm water and add a soothing, fragrant bath oil.

2

Let your body sink into the tub and soak the skin until it's completely softened (about 15 minutes).

3

Step out of the tub and sit down on a towel-covered chair, stool, or the toilet seat with the top down. Using your hands, gently rub the mineral salts all over your body, from your neck down to your feet (don't forget to get in between the toes!). Concentrate on the rough spots (elbows, knees, heels).

4

Step back into the tub and relax, allowing the salts to dissolve and the dead skin that has been exfoliated to slip away. While you're soaking (at least 20 to 30 minutes), take some time to read, do a crossword puzzle, brainstorm, or just enjoy the stillness. Add hot water to the tub as the temperature cools.

5

Once you've allowed yourself to relax and feel totally rested, it's time to step out of the bathtub, wrap yourself in a plush towel, and dry off slightly, leaving some moisture on your skin.

6

While the skin is still damp, apply some scented body cream.

7

Slip into your favorite pajamas, a slinky nightgown, or a comfy T-shirt and slippers and call it a night!

SCENT SAVVY

I think of fragrance as a little bit of luxury in a bottle. Some people are into oils; others prefer body splashes. I love sprays that smell like fruit, especially melon and mango scents. Ma used to say to me, "Why would you want to go around smelling like food?" But then she got a whiff of what I wear, and now she's addicted. The bottom line: Fragrance is all a matter of personal preference.

Before you decide on a signature scent:

Think about the message you want to convey—romantic, sporty, playful, confident, sexy, fun—and select a scent that says it.

Survey the array of choices available to you. Body splashes, for example, are lighter and less expensive than heavy perfumes.

After you find one:

Dab the scent on your pulse points—your neck, behind the ears, on the wrists, behind the knees. A spritz in the hair and between the breasts also has long-lasting effects.

Layering a scent—a bath oil, a body lotion, followed by a spray—increases its longevity.

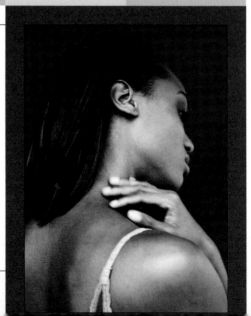

A CLASSIC
manicure

TOOLS

Emery board
Cuticle cream or lotion
A small bowl
A towel
Orange stick
Moisturizer or hand cream
Base coat
Nail color
Top coat

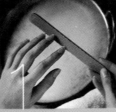

1 File each nail with the emery board to create the shape you want (oval, squared off, etc.). Do not drag the file back and forth; instead, use short strokes in one direction.

2 Apply cuticle cream to each nail and allow it to sink in for a few minutes, until the cuticles soften.

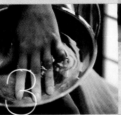
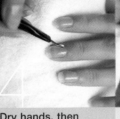
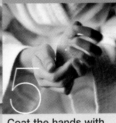

3 Soak your hands in a small bowl of warm water for at least 5 minutes, making sure all nails and cuticles are submerged.

4 Dry hands, then gently push back the cuticles. Do not cut the cuticles—you might risk infection or shred the cuticle.

5 Coat the hands with moisturizer and let it dry before applying nail polish.

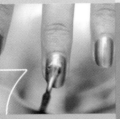

6 To prep the nails for color, polish them with a base coat. Paint one stroke down the middle, then apply another one on each side. Let dry.

7 Sweep on one coat of nail color, let that dry, then apply another.

8 As a finishing touch, layer on a clear top coat. The end result: Hands to die for!

BITING THE HANDS THAT FEED YOU

Nail biting is one nervous habit that's been hard for me to break. I still do it to this day. I'll be good for a while and leave my hands alone, and when I do, my nails get nice and healthy-looking. But then I'll be watching TV and start absentmindedly chomping away. And before you know it, I'm right back where I started.

As I've learned more about the effects of biting my nails, I've become more determined than ever to kick the habit. Nail biting can cause fungus and bacteria to grow around the nail beds, damaging them for good. If you're falling into the same pattern, why not stop now before the whole thing gets, well, uh, out of hand? These ideas, and a little willpower, should put you on your way:

Get regular manicures. Once you've forked over your own money to have your nails done, you'll be less likely to let that hard-earned handiwork go to waste.

Give your tastebuds a scare. Dip your fingertips into something distasteful, like vinegar or a bad-tasting nail coating made specifically for breaking this habit. Every time you put your hands in your mouth, you'll get an unpleasant surprise.

TOOLS

Foot tub
(or the bathtub will do
just fine)

Foot soak granules

A towel

Cuticle cream or lotion

Orange stick

Foot scrub

Pumice stone

Emery board

Cotton

Base coat

Nail color

Top coat

Nail polish remover

Moisturizer
or petroleum jelly

NEAT FEET

One thing I cannot stand is dirty feet. My house has hardwood floors and my feet are constantly sooty because I walk around barefoot, picking up dust and dirt. Sometimes when I'm really tired, I may skip a shower, but I will never fall into bed without washing my feet FIRST.

1 Fill a foot tub with warm water and pour foot soak granules into the water.

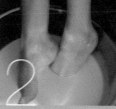

2 Soak feet for about five minutes to soften the skin.

3 Remove feet from water and apply a cuticle cream. Then, using an orange stick, gently push back the cuticles. (Don't force it, just apply pressure until the skin shifts back slightly.)

4 Apply foot scrub (or substitute an oatmeal scrub) to exfoliate the skin, and rinse off.

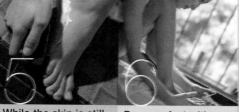

5 While the skin is still damp, use a pumice stone to lightly scrub thick areas like heels, the soles of the feet, and the bottom of the toes. (Never use a razor to scrape your feet—it could leave you open to infection.) Rinse away any residue.

6 Dry your feet with a towel, then clip nails if necessary and use the emery board to file them straight across (avoid rounded edges; they can cause ingrown toenails).

7 Place a ball of cotton in between each toe to spread them apart and catch any polish that might spill over.

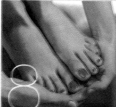

8 Starting with a clear base coat, paint one stripe up the middle, then one on each side.

9 Follow up with two coats of nail color, allowing for drying time in between each coat. Then finish off with a clear top coat.

10 When your nails are completely dry, put a tiny piece of cotton on top of the orange stick, dip it in nail polish remover, and wipe away any excess polish.

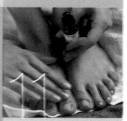

11 Slather on a moisturizing cream, or my favorite—petroleum jelly—to keep the footsies in top form!

The skin you're in is with you until the end, so it deserves to be treated with tender loving care. Nice wrapping makes a special package that's much more striking.

The first person who taught me about cosmetics was my mother, who is a makeup diva. She's been wearing makeup since she was a teen and has almost as many powders, eye shadows, and lipsticks as you'd find at any cosmetics counter. Long before I ever thought about wearing it, I used to sit in the bathroom and study every brush stroke of powder, eye shadow, and lipstick Ma applied as she "put on her face" in the morning. From my perch on the edge of the bathtub, I picked up a lot of pointers by watching her.

No doubt, the most important lesson she's passed on is that if you're going to wear makeup, you have to do it with precision.

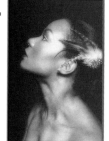

"Ma," Carolyn London

That sounds easy enough, but it's only easy if you know what you're doing. We've all seen too many women with makeup that's either overdone, underdone, or half done, and that doesn't do them any justice.

After years of practice, I think I've gotten the art of applying makeup (and it is an art form) down to a science, mainly because it's an essential part of my job. I have to wear makeup for fashion photo shoots, personal appearances, film, and television. And on those occasions, I can lay it on pretty thick, especially for high-fashion jobs. But that's all fantasy – what I want to talk about is real life.

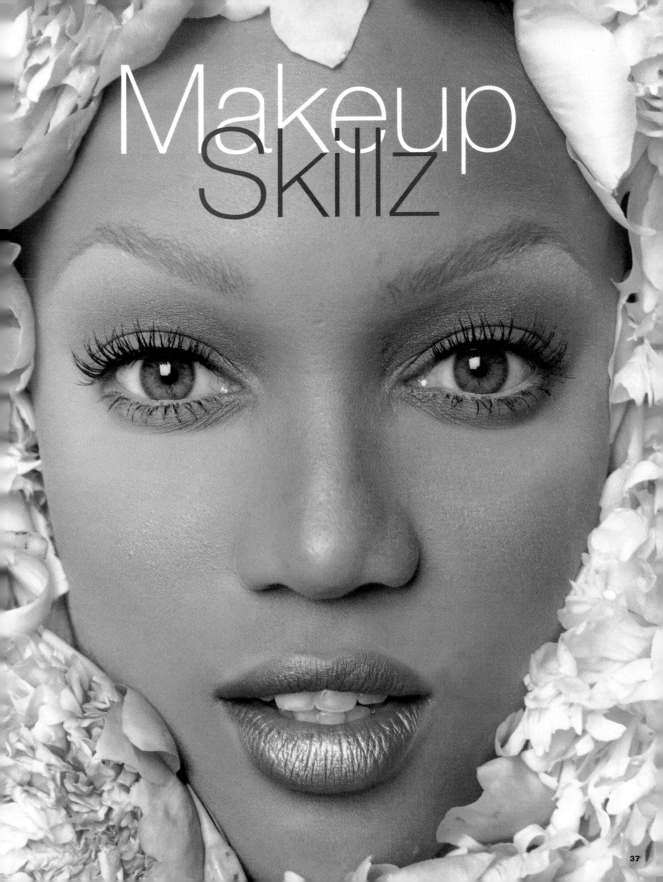

Makeup
Skillz

For Starters

I wasn't allowed to wear makeup outside the house until age thirteen, but that didn't stop me from dipping into my mother's makeup stash for a few practice sessions. Ma said it was okay to pile it on for fun and make-believe inside my bedroom—but I better not take my butt beyond the front doorstep. The one exception I remember was when I was nine years old and my

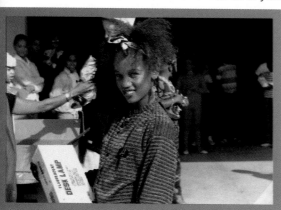

mother made me up as a punk rocker for Halloween— I won first prize (a desk lamp) for my costume!

There's a lot to be said for making your mistakes in the privacy of your own home. I can't even begin to count how many failed experiments I had along the way. The disasters I remember the most are the times I used to fill in my naturally arched eyebrows with so much black eyebrow pencil that I looked like Groucho Marx, and the time I wore the most ghastly shade of fluorescent green eye shadow because I thought I had to match my eye shadow to my emerald green

dress and my dyed-to-match green shoes. I don't have to tell you how horrible that looked. But, hey, at least I was color coordinated! Thank God for Ma—she gave me some honest feedback that kind of hurt my feelings but, in the long run, saved me a lot of embarrassment.

I saw a talk show not too long ago where the topic was young girls who were obsessed with makeup, and I was truly shocked to see so many girls under the age of fifteen with fully made-up faces. I mean, we're talking RuPaul—foundation, blush, lipstick, the works! Putting on that much makeup didn't do anything for them—except make them look old and hard. But in their minds they were the finest-looking things on the planet, and no one in the audience could tell them otherwise. The girls rattled off all kinds of weak reasons to explain why they needed so much makeup: "I don't have to please anybody but one person—and that's my boyfriend." "My makeup must be lookin' good because people stare at me all the time."

As you can probably guess, their mothers were not amused, especially when one of the girls said she was attracting guys twice her age. A lot of teen girls want to look older (I know, I was one of them), but there is plenty of time for that, and no need to rush. If you knew all the women I do who wish they had a youthful

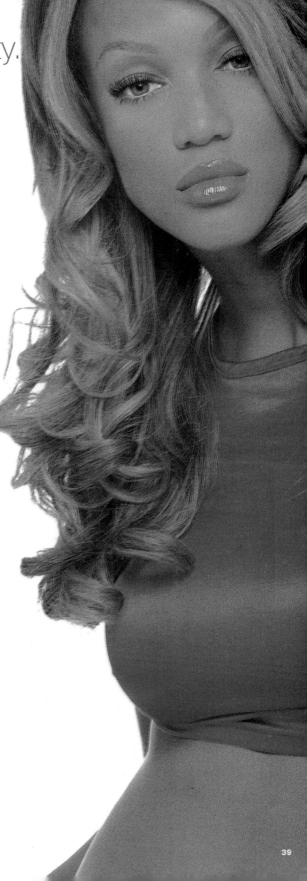

ot hide—our natural beauty.
s to "keep it real."

complexion so that they didn't have to wear any makeup at all, you'd understand why I recommend holding off on the full facial attack. Besides, I think the majority of guys find heavy makeup a turnoff. I guess they don't want any surprises.

I was thirteen when my mother lifted the makeup ban, but she was very specific about what I could wear. She even went with me to the neighborhood drugstore to help me pick it out. If she hadn't been there, I probably would have bought out the entire store (or at least as much as my allowance could get me). But she wasn't going for that! I came home with one mascara and some lip gloss—and both were clear, not one drop of color. I didn't care. I had my makeup on and you couldn't tell me anything because I just knew I looked good! Even though no one could actually see it, I knew it was there and that made me feel special.

I've added quite a few steps to my makeup routine since then—color included—but only after becoming more comfortable with what each product is for. Ready for a **crash course?**

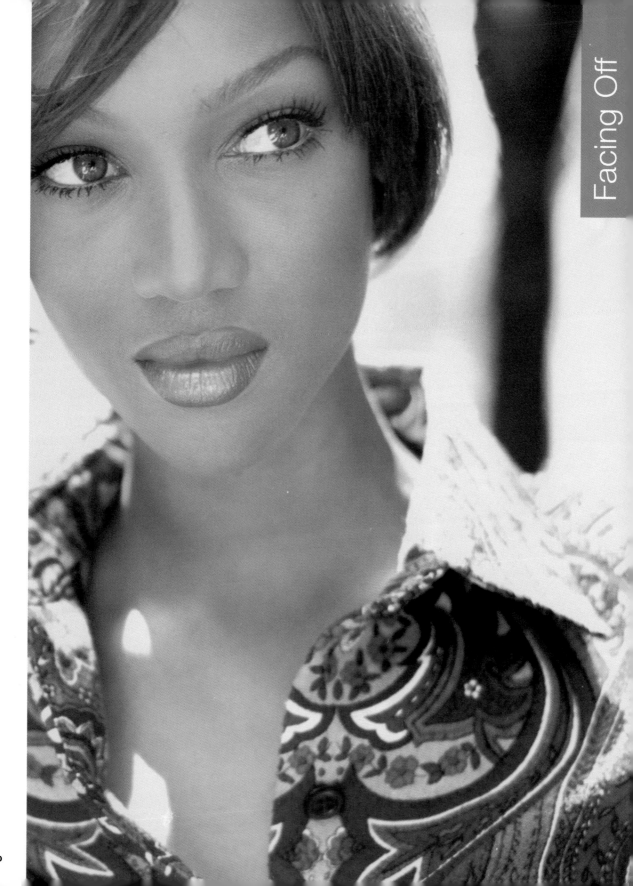

Learning how to apply makeup is like trying to perfect a new dance move–you've got to get all of the basic steps down first before you can move on to the flashy stuff. (I mean, it took me forever to learn how to do the butterfly, but once I got the hang of it, I learned how to do it on one leg, and even take it down to the ground!) **My advice: Read through this section a few times,** then set aside some time to "build your skillz." Practice with each product until you're comfortable with how to use it and how it looks on you. It's hard to know when enough is enough, especially when you're first starting out, so I suggest asking someone who you know will tell you straight-up whether or not you've gotten it right. With the information that follows, and plenty of practice, your makeup will look like it was done by a pro.

Whether it's a pimple, a birthmark, or a dark spot, most of us have something to hide. My nemesis is dark under-eye circles, which are hereditary in my family, and there's no way I'm ever going to get rid of them. That's where concealer comes in–it helps make slight imperfections virtually disappear.

Choosing it.

Typically, when you buy concealer, it doesn't come in as many shades as foundation does–the choices are usually either light, medium, or dark. I recommend using a color that is about one or two shades lighter than you are. Lightweight concealers are good for covering up marks such as blemishes and dark circles. Heavier versions work best on things like birthmarks and scars. Generally, you'd use concealer along with a foundation and pressed powder.

Using it.

The best way to hide dark under-eye circles is to apply concealer both on top of and slightly below the dark area. A lot of people make the mistake of using concealer only on top of the darkened area, and that's how they get that raccoon effect. Using your fingers or a sponge, blend in the concealer with a quick, dabbing motion, not a rubbing motion. The eye area has the thinnest skin on your face, so you have to treat it with extra care. The more you rub, the more you'll aggravate the skin (causing something almost like a bruise), and the darker your circles will appear.

If you're looking to hide a birthmark or pimple, lightly dab concealer on the blemish, then spread it out evenly so that it covers the blemish and some of the surrounding area. If you want to have a little fun, you can cover up the pimple with dark brown eyeliner. (Who knows–if the pimple is in the right place, you might get that Cindy Crawford look.)

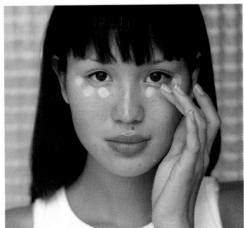

Concealer

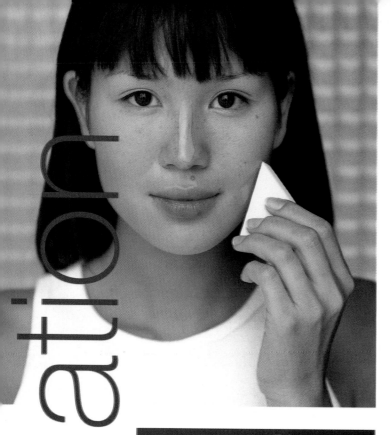

Foundation

Choosing it.

First, find a foundation that works with your skin type: oily, normal, or dry. Then try to match the color of the foundation to your undertones—an in-store makeup specialist can help you with this. Once you and the specialist have narrowed down the color choices, test the foundation on your jawline to see if it complements your undertones. (Be sure to wipe off the top of the foundation tester with a tissue first before you use it—you don't want somebody else's germs to wind up on your face.) One method I've found to be foolproof is to check how the foundation looks outside, in natural daylight. Most department stores don't mind if you do this. You'll know the color is right if it blends into your skin after it dries; ultimately, the color on your face should match your neck color. I mean, how many times have you seen someone whose foundation is so off she looks like she just saw a ghost, or just came from the tanning salon but only had her face done!

From personal experience, I know that it can be a real challenge, and sometimes very frustrating, to try to find a shade that precisely matches my skin tone. Fortunately, with so many cosmetics companies now expanding their lines to include a broader spectrum of shades, the chances of finding a foundation that matches are much better than they used to be.

If all else fails, you can borrow a trick from the pros and do some "custom blending" of your own. Buy two shades of foundation—one that is closest to your skin color, and one that is darker or lighter. Then mix them together, adding as much or

Foundation, or makeup base as it's also called, is applied after concealer. Some cosmetic companies have formulations for oily, normal, and dry skin. If it's done right, the look is like a second skin; it gives your face a smooth and even tone. Foundation can also protect your face from damaging sun rays as well as the dirt and air pollution that seeps into your pores throughout the day. But that doesn't mean you should lay it on thick. The only thing wearing a lot of foundation does is make you look like you have on a Halloween mask, and unless it's October 31, it's not appropriate. Remember: The idea is to let the real you show through.

as little of each color as you like until you get just the right shade. It's definitely not the cheapest or easiest process, but it may bring you closer to finding a shade that's right for you.

Using it.

I like to apply foundation with a triangular sponge because it lets me control how much or how little to put on, and where to put it. Most women—especially young women—don't need to use a lot of foundation, so I suggest squeezing a nickel-size blob of moisturizer into your hand, then adding foundation to it. This trick not only gives you a fresh, dewy look, but it also moisturizes your skin. (And, for the budget conscious, it's a great way to make the foundation last longer!)

Using the sponge, dot the foundation on your cheekbones, chin, nose, and forehead. Blend the foundation all the way into your hairline, over the ears, and under the chin. The idea is to even everything out—and I do mean everything!

Powder is usually applied after foundation to help set your make-up. But I sometimes prefer to use it instead of foundation, because it gets rid of shine and gives your face a finished appearance.

Choosing it.

Most powders come in either pressed or loose forms. I use both, but for different purposes. Loose powder is good for the initial at-home makeup application. Pressed powder is better for touch-ups, when

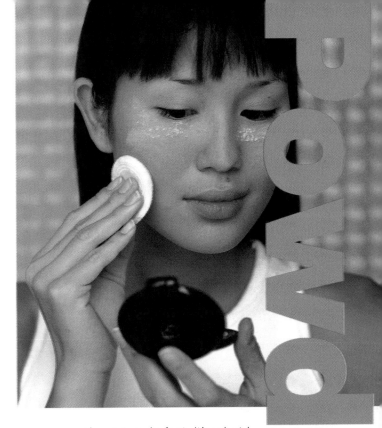

you are on the move. In fact, it's what I usually keep in my purse because I've had too many major messes in my handbag from carrying around loose powder that spilled all over everything.

Using it.

I think powder, whether pressed or loose, is best applied with a makeup brush. I prefer powder puffs for touch-ups. First, dip your brush or puff into the powder, then remove any excess by lightly blowing on the brush. If you want a lot of coverage, sweep the powder in broad strokes across your entire face and underneath your chin. If you want minimal coverage, apply the powder just to the areas on your face that tend to get shiny, such as the forehead, nose, and chin. If your skin is oily, you may need to reapply powder throughout the day to downplay the shine.

Blusher

When it's done right, blusher gives cheeks a healthy glow. A natural radiance is the look you should aim for.

Choosing it.

Blusher generally comes in cream or powder forms. I tend to use both, depending on the time of year. Cream blushers, which contain oil or moisturizers, are better for dry skin, especially in cold weather, because they add moisture to your skin. (But if you have sensitive skin, use caution—the additives in cream blusher can make you break out.) On the flip side, powders are much easier to manage than creams, because creams can look streaky if not applied correctly. Because I have dry skin, I like using cream blush when I'm not using any foundation. It blends into my skin better.

Using it.

First, smile at yourself in the mirror (go ahead and give yourself a big ol' grin—don't be shy), and find the round "apples" of your cheeks. This is where you should apply your blusher. Using clean, slightly damp fingers (if it's cream blush) or a blush brush (if it's powder blush), blend in the blush until your cheeks look slightly flushed. Here's where the control factor comes in. When in doubt, use a light touch—you can always go back and apply more. But if you start off with a heavy-handed approach, it's much harder to make corrections.

No makeup application would be complete without well-groomed eyebrows. Eyebrow filler enhances the shape of the brow, and fills in the blanks where the brows thin out.

Choosing it.

Eyebrow filler generally comes in pencil or powder form. But, quite frankly, I don't think you have to buy a product specifically for eyebrows. It's perfectly fine to use a dark eye shadow instead. In terms of shades, black is too harsh for most faces, even if your hair is jet black. A dark brown or blackish brown shade looks softer and more natural. There are also lighter colors for blondes and redheads.

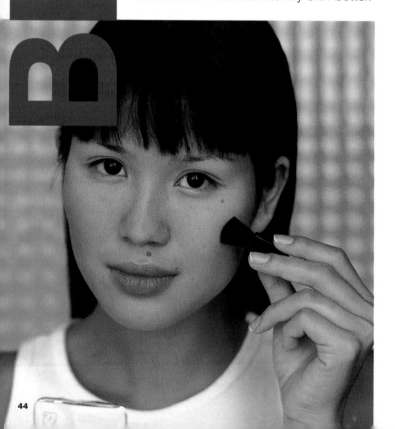

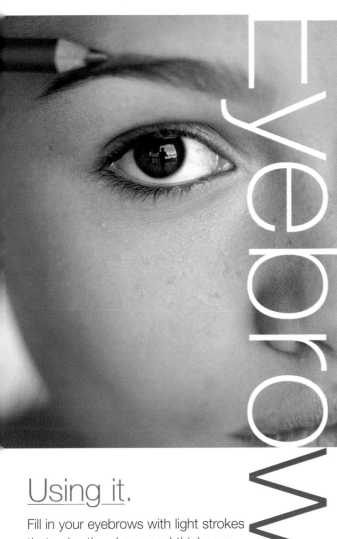

Eyebrow Filler

Using it.

Fill in your eyebrows with light strokes that echo the shape and thickness of your brows. The last thing you want is for your eyebrows to look drawn on. You don't have to fill in the entire brow. In fact, you shouldn't, because it will come off as looking too harsh. (Remember when I was talking about looking like Groucho?) Concentrate on the area closest to the bridge of your nose and the outer edges near the temples. Then blend the filler into your brows by brushing them (with an eyebrow brush or an extra toothbrush) in an upward motion, following the natural arch of the brow.

BROW TAMER TIME-SAVER

To whip unruly brows into shape, use clear mascara to brush them upward. I like to call clear mascara "eyebrow hair spray." It stiffens them in place with a hold that lasts all day.

the BROW BEAT

Because eyebrows frame the face, it is important to keep them neat. But pluck too much, and you can wind up looking like you're either in a constant state of surprise or perpetually angry. Unless your eyebrows are so bushy they actually meet in the middle, you don't really need to do a major plucking job.

Some tips:

Before you do anything, prep your skin for plucking by applying a warm washcloth to your eyebrows. I also recommend using some kind of soothing toner, like witch hazel, to clean the skin. If you don't clean the area first, you could get bumps or redness in the plucked area, which will take hours to fade away.

Always pluck your eyebrows in a diagonal direction, toward your ears.

Let the tail of your brows extend slightly past the outer corner of your eyes.

Don't go crazy. Tweeze a little at a time so that you don't take too much off at once. One major no-no is to pluck them into a shape that's really thick at the inner corners and super thin on the outside corners. Round half-moon shapes are another no-no. And of course you should never pluck them out completely. You've seen women do this—they pluck out their eyebrows, then draw in the shape they want. It's better—and more natural-looking—to work with what you've got.

How often you pluck depends on your hair-growth pattern. I think once or twice a week should be plenty. The key is to keep on top of the new growth, because if you don't, the hair will get too long and brows will lose their shape a lot quicker.

Plucking is way better than waxing, because you have more control over the amount of hair removal. If you make a mistake with wax, it will take your brows at least two weeks to grow back.

Last, but not least, never, ever shave your eyebrows. It can cause skin discoloration; plus, having a razor blade that close to your eyes simply isn't safe. Save the razor for your armpits and legs!

Eyeliner works sort of like a high-lighter pen – only instead of accenting the words on a page, the color accentuates your eyes. Most liners come in either liquid, felt-tip pen, or pencil form. Using eyeliner takes a steady hand. That's why I think pencil is the best to work with because it's easier to control – and easier to correct if you make a mistake.

Choosing it.

If you decide to use the pencil eyeliner, make sure its texture isn't too rough against your skin. (Some generic brands can be coarse and irritate the delicate skin around the eye.) You'll need a sharpener to keep the pencil tip in top form – the duller the tip, the less defined the line will be. Many products come with a sharpener in the package, but if the one you like doesn't happen to have one, any old pencil sharpener will do. Just don't use one sharpener for both purposes – you don't want to get pencil lead in your eyes or eyeliner smudges on your important papers.

A good brush is critical to using liquid eyeliner, so if you can, check out the tester before you make your purchase. The better the brush, the less difficult it will be to control the fluid. The other alternative: Buy an eyeliner brush separately. Another option is choosing a felt-tip liner, which is similar to buying a pen – if the color doesn't flow right away, give it a few good shakes. Then try it out on your hand to see if the thickness of the line is to your liking.

Using it.

Before you get started, make sure the pencil has a sharp point (but not so sharp that it could put out an eye). Then dab the pencil on the back of your hand to soften the point slightly. Holding the eyeliner as you would hold a number 2 pencil, start by drawing a line along the outer rim of your top eyelid, directly above the eyelashes. Repeat this step along the outer rim of your lower lid, below the eyelashes. (This isn't easy, because you're dealing with loose, flexible skin, which makes it harder to control the application, not to mention that your eye-lashes can get in the way. I still have trouble drawing a straight line, and I even know makeup pros who make crooked lines.) As you do this, pull the outer corner of the eye slightly taut to make the skin as smooth as possible. I prefer using eyeliner on the outside rims because it's safer. Lining the inner rim might give you a more dramatic look, but there's also the chance that some traces of eyeliner might remain in your eye after you remove your makeup. Rather than risk an allergic reaction, it's better to line the outer rims. Last, smudge the lines a little with a sponge applicator or finger for a softer look. (It's also a good way to camouflage your mistakes if the lines you drew weren't all that neat.)

For liquid eyeliner, dip the tip of the brush into the fluid until it is slightly wet. You may want to test the thickness of the line on the back of your hand before you apply it to your eyes. Then follow the same directions as above, with the exception of smudging the line. Felt-tip pen users should follow suit.

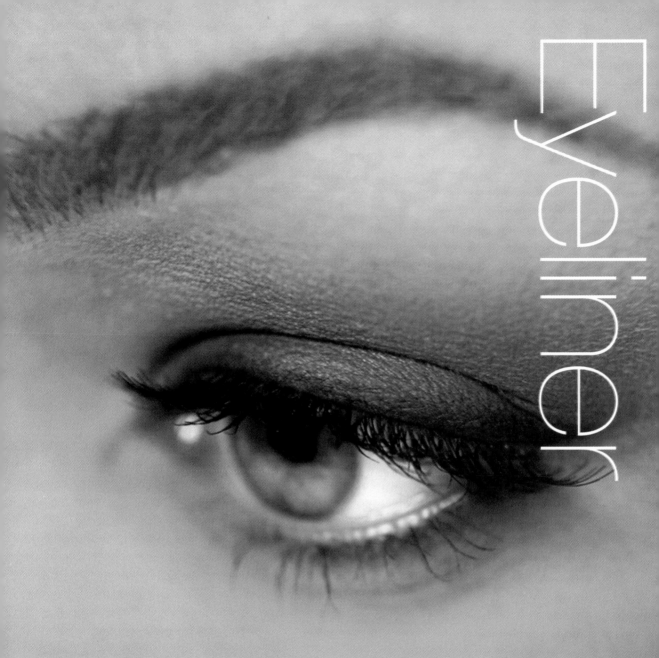

Eyeliner

Eye shadow is the icing on the cake as far as I'm concerned. Your makeup will look fine without it, but it adds that extra flavor. I love to experiment with a range of colors. With every mix and match, I'm able to give my eyes a different look. I've picked up many of my methods from the professional makeup artists who deal with it every day. They tell me that eye shadow is the most complicated makeup to apply because, in order to do it right, you usually need at least two different shades—one to go on the eyelid and a lighter one to wear on the brow bone.

Choosing it.

Eye shadows come in cream, pencil, and powder form. Creams go on smoothly, but tend to crease in the corners. Some people prefer to use pencil, but it can be rough on the skin around the eye. Powders, my personal favorite, are less complicated. The only danger here is that it's easy to go overboard if you don't use a light touch.

As for color choice, I say try them all! No color is off-limits! Yes, even vibrant shades are fine, as long as you use them in moderation. It's all about how you apply it. What I like to do when I think a color is too bright is to layer a neutral color, like a soft brown, over it. It helps to tone down the color.

Using it.

Until you become really skilled at this, keep things simple by sticking to one neutral shade, such as a soft brown or smoky gray, and one slightly lighter shade, like a beige or sand, to use as a highlighter. Using an eye shadow brush or sponge applicator, sweep the darker color across the lid, just under the brow bone. Then apply the lighter shade above that on the brow bone, extending it outward toward the temples.

Contrary to popular belief, you don't have to match your eye shadow to your outfit. In fact, it's better not to coordinate colors this way. (Remember my green on green on green experience?) You want people to notice your face, not how your face blends in with your beautiful clothes. Each should be separate and have a life of its own.

One way to make the most of your makeup dollars is to use a darker eye shadow as an eyeliner. Using a sponge applicator, draw the shadow across the outer rim of the lids, close to your lashes, just as I mentioned earlier, then smudge. It's a gentler and softer way to achieve eye definition.

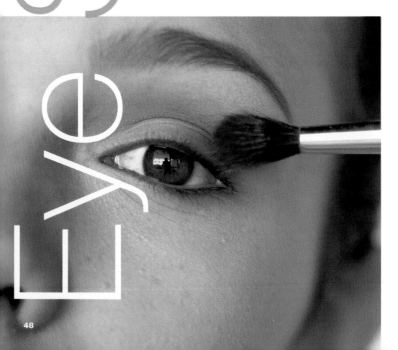

Even when I'm in a rush, I rarely leave the house without a couple of quick coats of mascara. Not only does it add color, but it also calls attention to your eyes by making lashes look thicker and longer. In my opinion, black and brown are the best colors for all women. If your hair is blond or light brown, brown mascara is a better choice because it looks more natural. I prefer to use black mascara because I have very thin lashes and brown just doesn't bring them out enough, but you should choose whichever color is most flattering on you.

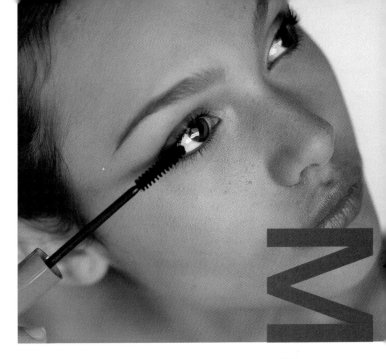

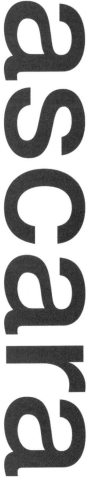

Choosing it.

Look for mascara that goes on smoothly, without flaking or causing your lashes to clump together. The brush you choose has a lot to do with that. Wide spaces between the bristles encourage clumps; a brush with narrowly spaced bristles minimizes the chances of this happening. A picture on the package or an in-store tester will show you what kind of brush you're getting before you buy it.

If you're trying to decide between regular and waterproof mascara, remember that the more waterproof the product, the harder it will be to remove. On the plus side, waterproof mascara isn't as likely to run—something to keep in mind if you play sports or wear contact lenses. (By the way, you should always put your contacts in first, before you put on any makeup.)

Whatever you do, don't try on mascara from the samples at the cosmetics counter. I once got a bad case of pink

eye (or to be technical, conjunctivitis) from doing just that—and believe me, that's one experience I don't ever want to experience again. I walked around for a week with swollen, crusty, tearing eyes.

If you want to try out the color before you put down the dollars, ask a salesperson if there is an unopened sample you can use, or just buy the least expensive mascara you can find until you hit on the one that works for you. Since harmful bacteria is likely to hide out in mascara, you should plan to discard the old tube and buy a new one every three months. It will cost you, but it's worth it if you want healthy eyes.

Using it.

When you first pull the brush out of the tube, take a tissue and wipe off any excess mascara—this eliminates those thick blobs you sometimes get when the mascara is brand-new. Start the brush close to your eyelid (watch that you don't get any in your eye), then sweep it

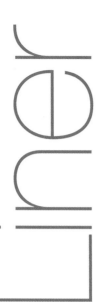

Lip Liner

outward toward the tips of your lashes. Take your time—I've seen women (myself included) stab themselves in the eye with the brush too many times to rush through this step. Mascara can be a difficult product to use if you're not experienced. It takes a sure hand, a sharp eye, and lots of practice.

I like to apply mascara to both the top and bottom lashes because it makes the eyes look larger and perkier. One coat is plenty for everyday wear, but if you're looking for a little more definition, you can layer on a few coats. Just make sure you allow enough time for your lashes to dry a little between each coat; otherwise, you'll end up with a clumpy mess!

If, after all this careful application, you still wind up with thick clumps, take a small toothbrush or eyelash comb and brush them out, making sure that none of the excess mascara flakes off into your eyes. Another neat trick: To avoid getting stray mascara marks on your eyelids, try not to open your eyes too wide while applying.

Lip liners (or lip pencils) accentuate the shape of your lips and keep lipstick from bleeding or running outside your natural lip line. They can also help your lipstick last longer.

Choosing it.

Lip liner is supposed to blend in with your lipstick, not stand out as a separate entity. So when making a selection, choose a color that is either the same or no more than two shades darker than your lipstick. The pencil texture should be soft enough to glide on smoothly, but not so soft that it makes sloppy lines. On the other hand, if the texture is too dry, it will make your lips feel likewise. Try to find one that strikes a good balance.

Using it.

Draw a thin line along the edge of your top and bottom lip. Then, after you apply your lipstick, blend both together until you can't tell where your lip liner ends and the lipstick begins. If your lipstick has a tendency to wear out long before the day is over, you can also use lip liner as a primer before you apply your lipstick. Just fill in a thin coat all over the lips, then apply lipstick on top of the liner.

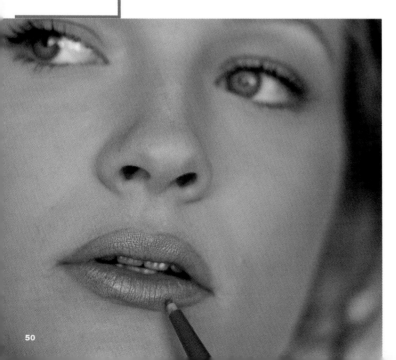

Lipstick is one makeup product almost every woman can count among her favorites. Lipstick or lip gloss gives the face an instant lift, and they both can also serve a practical purpose: keeping lips moisturized. (We all know there's nothing worse than dry, chapped lips!)

A lot of women feel self-conscious about their full lips. But in recent years they've become very desirable, so don't let anyone tell you differently. I know a lot of women who have spent a fortune trying to plump theirs up with cosmetic surgery, so if you are blessed with full lips, make the most of them.

Choosing it.

To tell you the truth, I prefer flavored lip gloss to any kind of lipstick. Sometimes people say, "Tyra, that shiny lip gloss look went out years ago," but I like it and I'm gonna keep on wearing it. When I was younger my friends and I bought every flavor, from watermelon and strawberry to bubble gum, and I guess I haven't outgrown that. I still wear it and I still love it. That's the same criteria you should use when you make your choices. Wear what you like. If you want a look that's a little more sophisticated, you can always layer on lip gloss over lipstick.

I don't believe in lipstick rules. It's one product you can go crazy with, so don't ever feel that your skin color is too dark to wear something on the pale side or too fair to wear something bright. Just have fun!

And just another reminder about testers: I know I said this before, but it bears repeating—**beware of in-store testers.** You don't know whose lips have touched them before yours. Ask for an individual sample instead. If there aren't any samples available, try out this trick that I picked up at a cosmetics counter. Ask the salesperson if she keeps alcohol at the counter, and, if so, have her disinfect the tip of the tester with alcohol, then wipe off the tester with a tissue before you try it out.

If there's no alcohol around, your best bet is to test the color on the back of your hand, then put your hand close to your face to see how the color looks close to your lips. It's not perfect, but it's safer than putting it directly on your lips.

Using it.

Using a lip brush is a good way to stay within the lip lines, make colors look more vibrant, and help lipstick to stay on longer. It also prevents you from putting

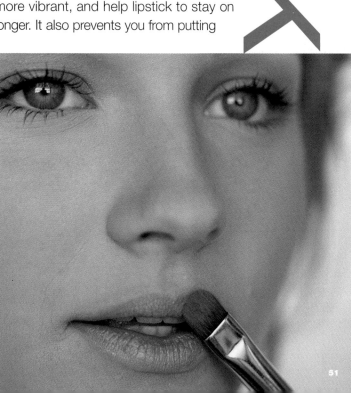

Lips

on too much lipstick because it allows you to control how much you apply. Although I have a friend who can apply lipstick perfectly, straight from the tube without using a mirror, I haven't quite reached that level of expertise, so I use a lipstick brush and a mirror every time.

Starting in the middle of your bottom lip, follow your lip line and draw the lipstick outward to each corner. Repeat on the top lip. Do not smack your lips together. This tends to make lipstick go outside your lip line. If you happen to go outside the lines, just take a Q-Tip and remove the excess. Then fill in the middle, giving even coverage to the top and bottom lips.

The last step is to check the intensity. If you think the color is too strong, take it down a bit by blotting your lips with a tissue until the color looks more natural.

For Your **LIPS** *ONLY!*

Lipstick is made for lips—not for cheeks—so don't try to cut corners by using your lipstick as a blusher. It can lead to breakouts. I know, because I've tried it before, when I ran out of blusher. All I wound up with was a face full of pimples!

Brushing**UP**

A basic set should include:

If you can afford it, it's worth it to invest in a good set of professional makeup brushes. Brushes enhance the quality of your makeup job. I find that I use less makeup when I'm using good brushes, and my makeup lasts longer—which means the money in my wallet lasts longer too.

powder brush
blush brush
lip brush
eye shadow brush
eyeliner brush

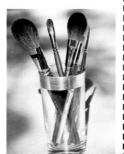

Falsies
for Your Eyes

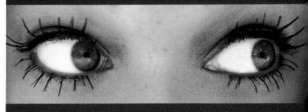

False eyelashes give your eyes a wide-eyed, innocent look. Some people think they make you look sexier, but if applied correctly, I think they can make you look sweeter. False eyelashes are time-consuming to apply, so I recommend reserving them for special occasions. It takes practice, practice, practice to put them on perfectly!

A FEW GUIDELINES:

Look for the softest, most natural-looking false eyelashes you can find—avoid those big, thick ones that look like wings.

Before you attach the eyelashes, try them on for size on top of your existing lashes.

Use either clear-colored or black glue to apply them. I prefer black glue because it looks like eyeliner and camouflages the area where the lashes are attached. Apply a thin strand of glue along the base of the false eyelash.

Using blunt tweezers or your fingers, attach the lashes to your eyelid slightly above your real lashes. If you apply them directly on top, they will get all tangled up, or, worse, glued together.

Once you've gotten them attached, use your fingers to blend the false eyelashes into your own real lashes. Most people don't do this, which makes it very obvious that the lashes are fake.

Always use makeup remover to detach the false eyelashes. Even though it will probably destroy the lashes, it will save your own. If you try to remove them without using some kind of solvent, you might pull out some of your real eyelashes. The one time I didn't use any remover, I went around with barely any lashes at all. That was the year the glamour look was in—big hair and tons of makeup—and every makeup artist was using false eyelashes. Some of them would recycle them. They'd just rip them right off you and use them on someone else.

Learning how to apply false eyelashes does take some time, so don't let it get to you if you mess up on the first couple of tries. Eventually, you'll get the hang of it.

Lashing Out

If you're not ready for false eyelashes, using an eyelash curler can give you almost the same effect. Eyelash curlers press your lashes into a curlier shape, and make eyes look more alert and happy. But they can cause problems if used incorrectly. A few precautions:

When you slide the curler over your top lashes, don't close the clamps completely at first—you want to make sure there's no skin caught in the opening, just lashes. Gradually add more pressure, but never go full force.

Be careful that your eyelid doesn't get caught in the crimper. You haven't felt real pain until you've had two metal bars clamping down on your sensitive eyelids. *OUCH!*

Remember to apply mascara after you use the curler, and not before, because the mascara can stick to the curler and pull out your lashes.

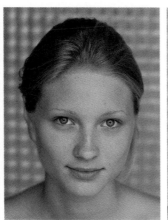
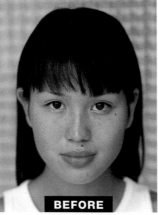
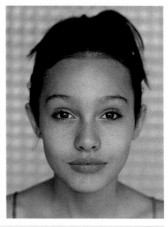

BEFORE

AFTER

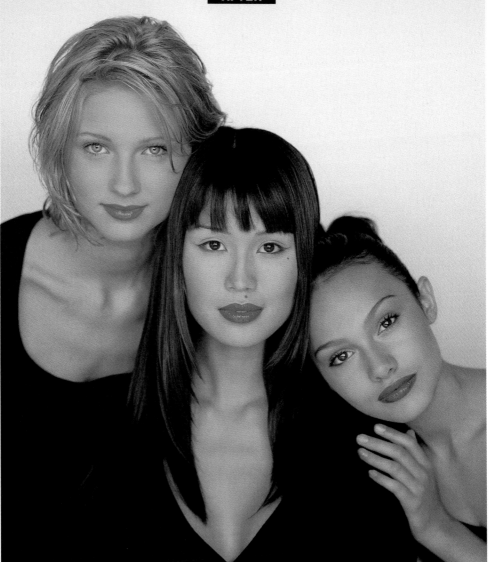

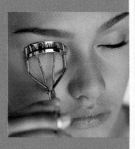

Easy Makeup Looks for **Day** and **Night**

Now that you've found the makeup you want in the colors you like, I thought I'd let you in on a few ways to keep your mirror time to a minimum. Who wants to be sitting in front of a makeup mirror for hours? I mean, I know you have places to go, people to see, things to do…

Unless I'm working, I don't wear makeup every day, mainly because I'm too lazy to put it on. But when I do wear it, it always makes me feel polished and pulled together. I have two routines that I go through, one for daytime and one for those nights when I'm going somewhere special and really want to make a statement. I've outlined each below. You can follow them step by step, or just pull out the pieces that work best for you.

DAYTIME POLISH

1. To mask my dark circles, I start with a few sweeps of concealer.

2. I usually pass on wearing foundation, and instead just dust some pressed powder on my t-zone (forehead, nose, and chin).

3. Cream blush comes next. I dot some on the apples of my cheeks and blend in well.

4. I don't go many places without my mascara. My lashes are very thin, so I like to put on at least two coats or more.

5. Last, I glide on some lip gloss.

The entire process takes me about **five minutes!**

EVENING DRAMA

I guess you could say I'm kind of a bum most of the time, but sometimes my friends will say, "Tyra, we're going out to dinner tonight so don't wear sweats and puh-lease put some makeup on your face, girl!" So for those special occasions, I allow myself a lot more time for my makeup. I don't go all out–I save that look for fashion shoots, movie premieres, and any other personal appearances I have to make–but just this little bit of extra effort always makes me feel special.

1. I start with my dark circles, dotting concealer first until I'm well-covered, then I apply my foundation.

2. Next, I use loose powder to set the foundation.

3. Eyebrows are up next. Because mine are so far apart, I use an eyebrow pencil to fill them in a little closer together, then extend the ends of them slightly.

4. To give me a healthy glow, I brush on some peach-tone powder blush.

5. Eyeliner puts my eyes into focus.

6. I apply a smoky eye shadow for a sultry effect.

7. Evening calls for something extra, and for me, that means false eyelashes.

8. At night, I like to wear darker, richer lipstick shades. After I line my lips with a lip pencil, I fill them in with lipstick and blot with a tissue.

9. And, of course, I end with a couple of layers of lip gloss!

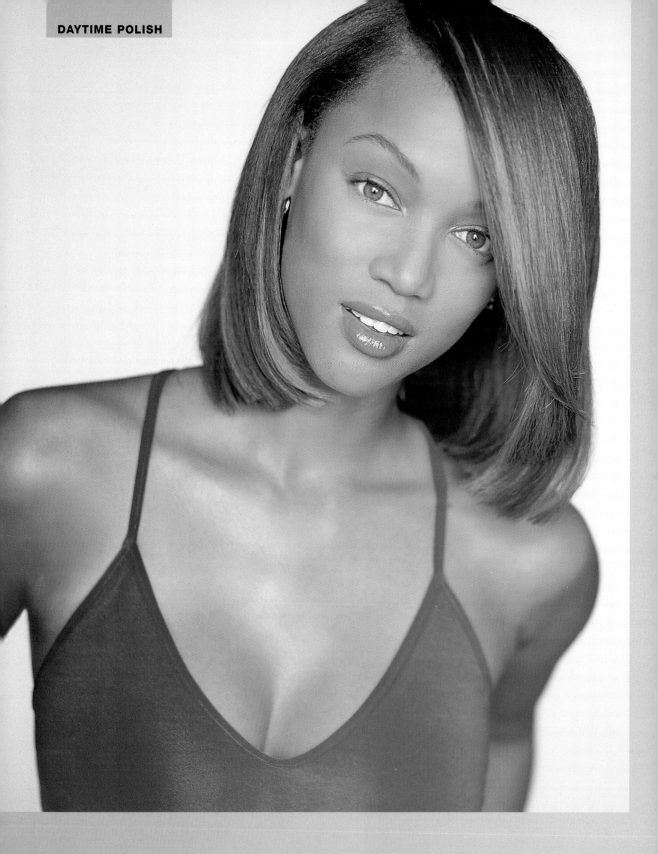

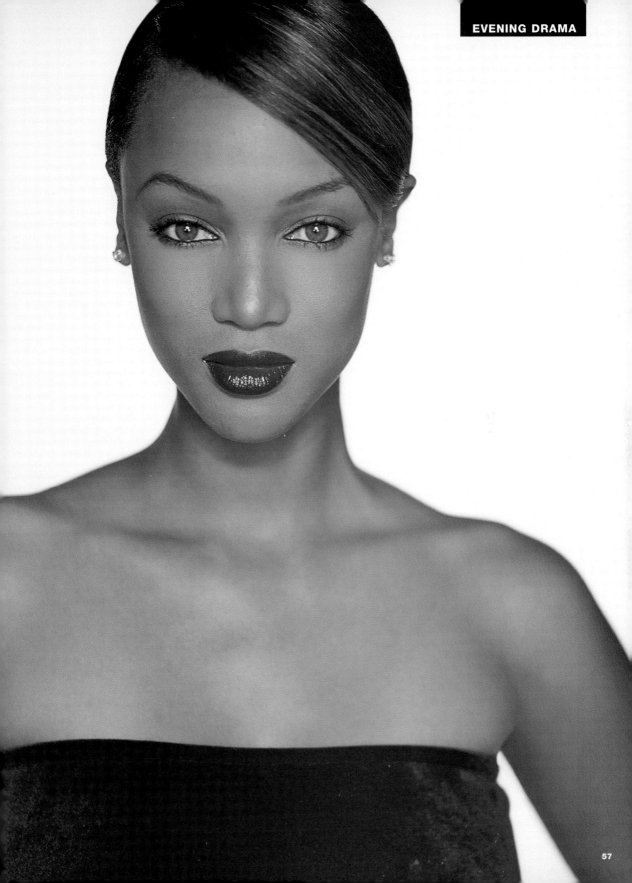

Kiss your **ASH** Goodbye

Until recently it was almost impossible for women of color to find foundation that matched their skin tones (it usually ended up looking ashy). But cosmetic companies finally caught on and they now produce makeup for *every* skin tone–from the lightest to the darkest, and every shade in between. **Thank goodness!**

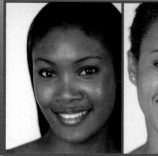 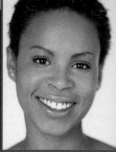 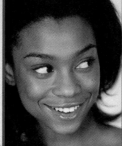

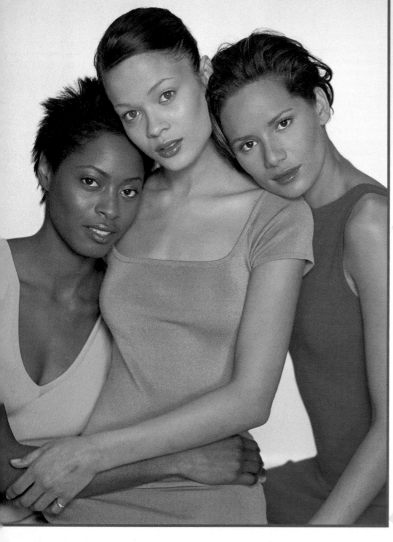

Good Light
Will Do You Right

Doing your makeup in the same lighting you'll be seen in during the day minimizes mistakes (like putting on more than you need). I always do my daytime makeup in natural light. I have a table that faces a window, and this gives me the best, even light so that I can see every little thing I'm doing.

One thing to watch out for: **shadows.** They can trick you into believing that you didn't cover a spot when you've actually gone over it at least two or three times. A good way to make sure your makeup is just right: Invest in one of those makeup mirrors that has a choice of lighting options. I think it's worth the money just to make sure you don't overdo it. Plus, if you want to apply your makeup at night, the natural daylight thing just ain't gonna work.

Five Makeup No-Nos

1. Community Makeup
No one should ever share makeup, especially mascara, lipstick, and eyeliner.

Once, during the fashion shows, one of the models had pink eye, and since the makeup artist didn't know it, he used the same mascara on the other girls. By the end of the week, we were all walking around with red, sickly eyes.

2. Lethal Lip Liner
It's okay to go a shade darker, but not four, five, or six shades darker.

3. Fake-Looking Foundation
Foundation should match the skin tone perfectly. Save the mask for masquerade parties!

4. Groucho Brows
Eyebrow filler should be handled with a light touch.

5. Bad Blending
If the makeup application isn't flawless, what people will notice when they see you is a lot of unflattering lines and colors.

I f I ever had to suddenly stop modeling, I know I could always get a job as a professional makeup artist. When I first started in the business, I had to do my own makeup at the fashion shows because whenever I would stand in line for the best makeup artists, I'd always get pushed aside by some supermodel who felt she didn't have to wait. (It's funny, but some of those same models would see the makeup job I did on myself and ask me to do theirs! I told them they should have thought about that before they jumped ahead of me in line!) I had learned so much from watching Ma and practicing with different looks at home that I knew exactly what to do at a fashion show. I would just run backstage shouting, "Okay, what's the look we're going for?" and then get to work.

As I've gained more experience in the industry, I've had the opportunity to work with some of the most talented makeup artists in the business. Four of my favorites are Fran Cooper, Sam Fine, Billy B., and Troy Jensen. I worked with Fran for the first time on a photo shoot for *Elle* magazine. Sam and I met on some bogus job that didn't turn out to be much of anything, but we became great friends. Billy B. did the makeup for my milk ad, and Troy did my makeup for the first music video I was in.

Since all four understand my face better than I do, I asked them if they would share some of their makeup philosophies with you. They were more than happy to:

Fran Cooper: "It is important to think about makeup in terms of situation and mood. Adjust the look so that it is appropriate for the time and season—summer, winter, day, or evening. It's also important to be versatile. People can get caught up in the same thing. It's better to change your look from time to time."

Sam Fine: "Fine-tuning is what makes the difference between okay makeup and great makeup. It enhances what is already there, making sure that everything is perfect. That means giving a little extra attention, care, and love to certain aspects of the face, like white eyeliner carefully applied to the inner rim of eyelids to make your eyes look brighter, adding an extra coat of mascara, or using foundation on a wedge sponge around your mouth to make sure lipstick and lip liner are perfect. Fine-tuning gives you a face that's finished and precise."

Billy B.: "Much like she would do with clothing, a woman should find the makeup that works for her and use it to create a wardrobe of basic colors, such as a good palette of neutrals. Then she can update here and there with something seasonal. Not every trend is for everybody. Evaluate them all and pick the one that best suits you—something that makes you feel good."

Troy Jensen: "Makeup is not always about making someone look made-up or beautiful. Many times it is about inventing something different and unusual. Part of the creative process is incorporating texture by using various elements such as beads, feathers, glitter, jewels, stencils, and body paints that enable you to create a desired image. Instead of the makeup application being a 'makeover,' think of it as a crafted project."

To give you a better idea of the kind of magic these guys can work, I've included two pictures of me, one before and one after a makeup sitting. In the "before" picture, I've marked off all the things the makeup artists will correct in the "after" photo. It's amazing what a little makeup and photo retouching can do. It just goes to show you that you can't believe everything you see in the magazines. I hope it makes you feel a bit better about measuring up to us models, because most of the look comes straight out of a bottle.

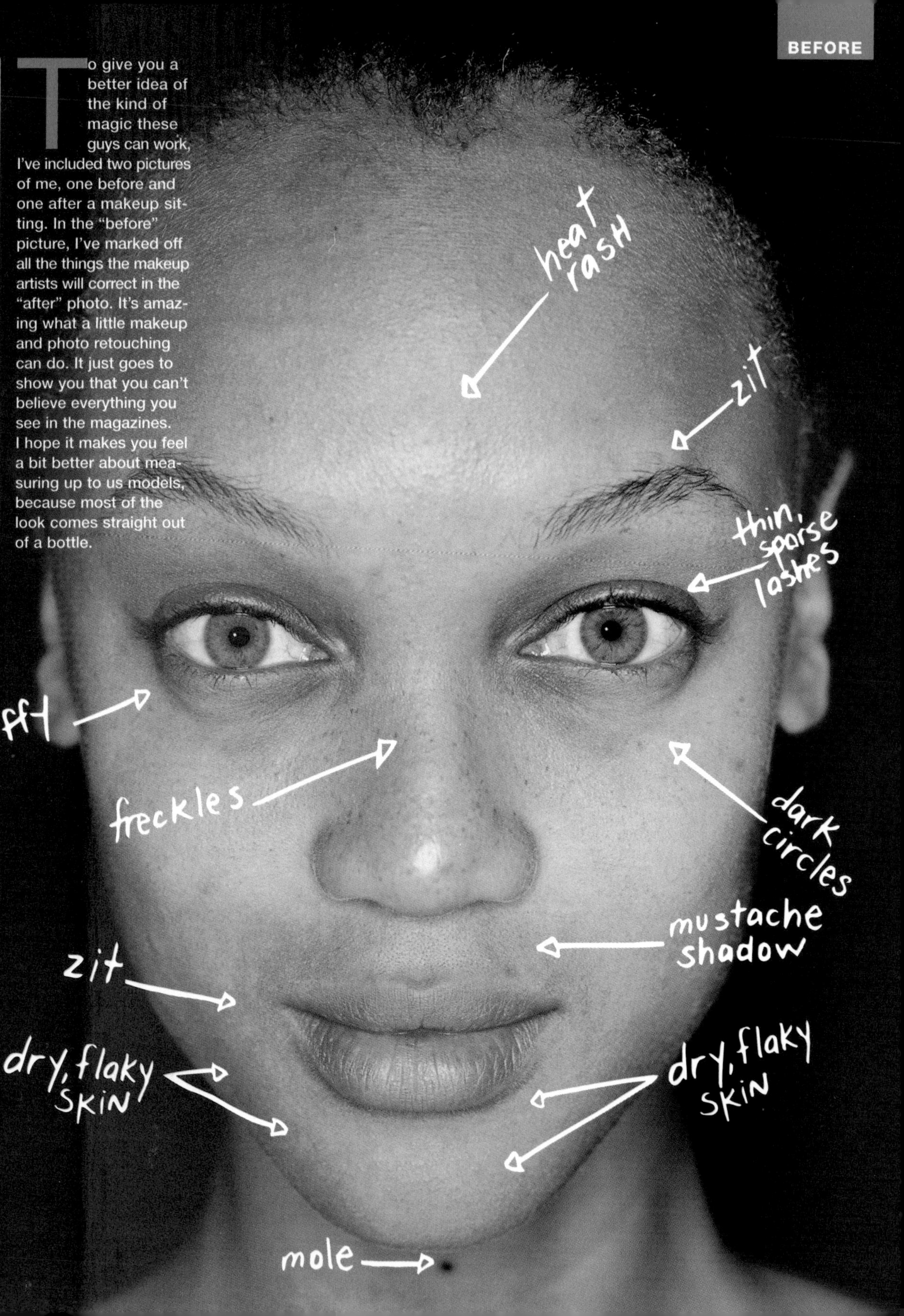

heat rash

zit

thin, sparse lashes

puffy

freckles

dark circles

mustache shadow

zit

dry, flaky skin

dry, flaky skin

mole

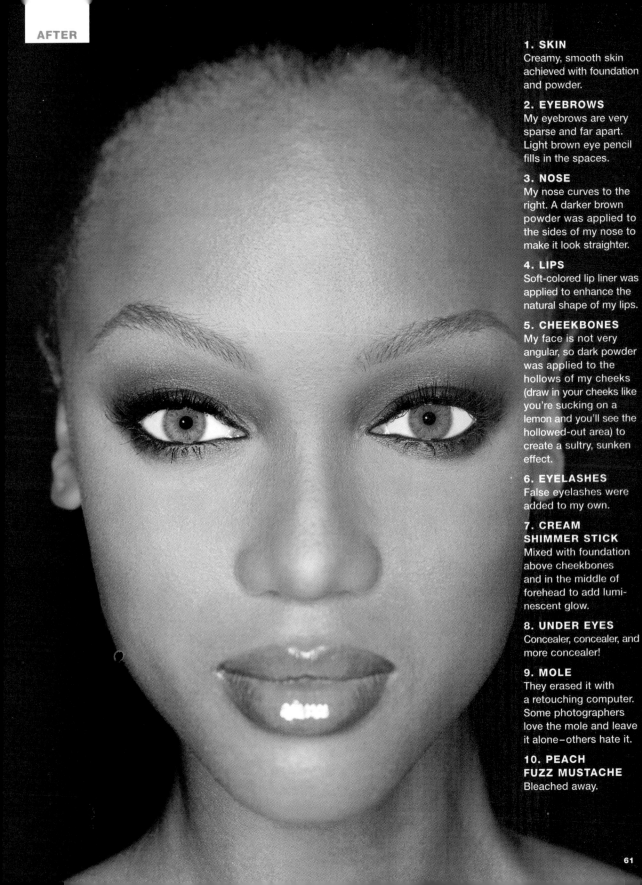

1. SKIN
Creamy, smooth skin achieved with foundation and powder.

2. EYEBROWS
My eyebrows are very sparse and far apart. Light brown eye pencil fills in the spaces.

3. NOSE
My nose curves to the right. A darker brown powder was applied to the sides of my nose to make it look straighter.

4. LIPS
Soft-colored lip liner was applied to enhance the natural shape of my lips.

5. CHEEKBONES
My face is not very angular, so dark powder was applied to the hollows of my cheeks (draw in your cheeks like you're sucking on a lemon and you'll see the hollowed-out area) to create a sultry, sunken effect.

6. EYELASHES
False eyelashes were added to my own.

7. CREAM SHIMMER STICK
Mixed with foundation above cheekbones and in the middle of forehead to add luminescent glow.

8. UNDER EYES
Concealer, concealer, and more concealer!

9. MOLE
They erased it with a retouching computer. Some photographers love the mole and leave it alone—others hate it.

10. PEACH FUZZ MUSTACHE
Bleached away.

Crazy
Face

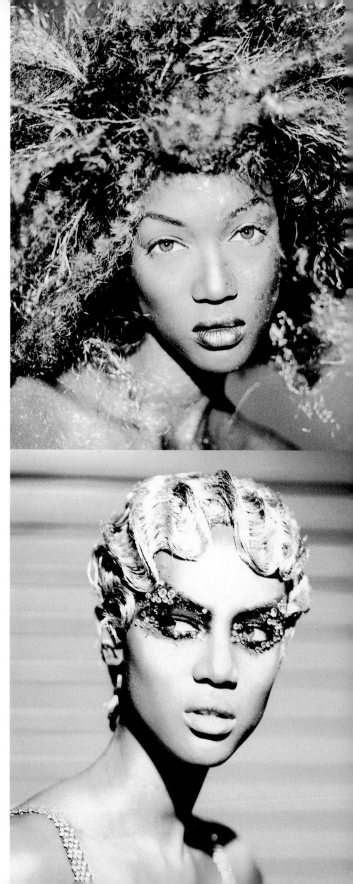

When I first started working with Troy and wanted to expand my makeup options, he suggested that I study the makeup looks I liked in fashion magazines and try to re-create them. He says that although the images may look insane, there is always something to learn from even the most outrageous creations. It's all about stretching the imagination. We may see a model whose makeup looks like she's going to a wild masquerade party and think, "That is too weird for me," or "Where would I ever wear that?" But the intention is not for you to copy the look brush stroke for brush stroke. It's to inspire you. If you take a few minutes to look beyond the zaniness, there's probably at least one neat trick or two that you can adapt to your own style.

That's what Troy and I hope the creations in these photographs will inspire you to do. We had a lot of fun (and I went through a little torture) creating each of them, using different textures to produce looks that are way out of the norm. "I really didn't know what I was going to do at first," says Troy. "I just looked at the materials I had in front of me and ran with it." And boy did he run with it!

Troy: "For this photo, I wanted Tyra to look like a live sculpture. So first I painted her entire body in milk chocolate body makeup. Then I took a paintbrush and splattered her with liquid gold metallic body paint. To interpret this look, you might want to just use a little touch here and there. Who's to say what's gaudy and what's not? It's all a matter of what you like."

Tyra: "What I like about this look is that you can take the gold idea and decide maybe I'll use some gold eye shadow on my brow bone, or a layer of golden blush or lip gloss over another color to add some shimmer."

Rhinestone Cowgirl >

Troy: "A lot of times when I travel, I see a street style, like women imitating a Gwen Stefani look by wearing the gemstones in the middle of their forehead, and it's very creative. Here in the States, we tend to wait for something to become a trend before we try it out. I say, be adventurous!"

Tyra: "Maybe you could put a small rhinestone where a mole would be. Obviously there's a time and a place for everything, and you wouldn't want to wear this look to school or to the office. But to a party or a club, why not?"

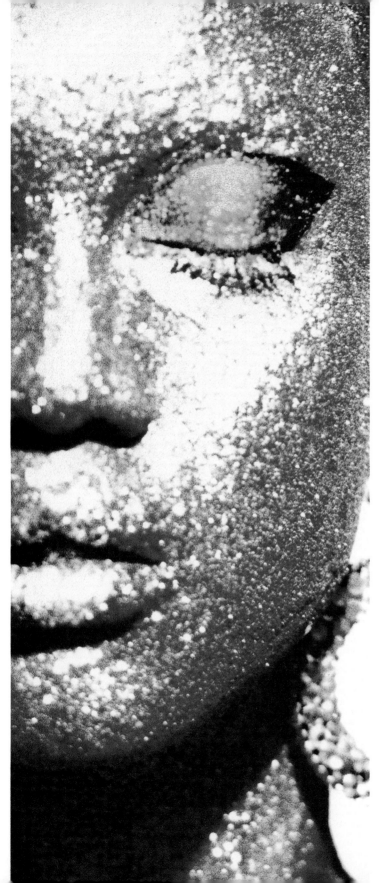

Troy: "Glitter isn't something that people normally add to their makeup regimen. But for night you could add a little shine to the lips or to the eyes, just as accents. You don't have to go over the top."

Tyra: "This was probably the hardest shot to sit through because Troy had to keep reapplying the glitter. Weeks later, I still kept finding glitter everywhere. I was also miserable because the glitter hardened like a mask and sort of paralyzed my face. Thank goodness the photo came out pretty cool because I would have been pissed to go through such torture for a messed-up outcome. I like how the look turned out, but if I ever see Troy coming at me with a bag full of pink glitter again, I'm outta there."

Looking through magazines for inspiration has worked well for me. If I'm going to a major event and want my look to have drama, but Troy, Sam, Billy, or Fran are unavailable, I can do it myself. My only words of caution: I always make sure I start practicing with an idea long before the day of the event, when I know no one will see me. That way, if I get it wrong, it doesn't set me in a panic when I have to take it all off and start over.

Tyra's **Top-Ten Makeup** Faves

- - - - - - - -

1. CONCEALER
Keeps my dark circles undercover.

2. PRESSED POWDER
Controls that greasy shine.

3. PEACH BLUSHER
Always makes me look fresh and energetic, even when I'm not.

4. DARK BROWN EYE SHADOW
Adds mystery to my eyes.

5. CREAM SHIMMER STICK
Gives me that radiant glow.

6. BLACK MASCARA
I love to pile it on!

7. DEEP BROWN CONTOUR POWDER
Gives me the cheekbones I wasn't born with.

8. DARK BROWN EYELINER
One touch changes pimples into moles.

9. FALSE EYELASHES
I love that wide-eyed doe look!

10. FLAVORED LIP GLOSS
Tastes as good as it looks.

I've come a long way from playing with my mother's makeup. Today, I play with my own! **Now it's YOUR turn.**

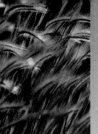

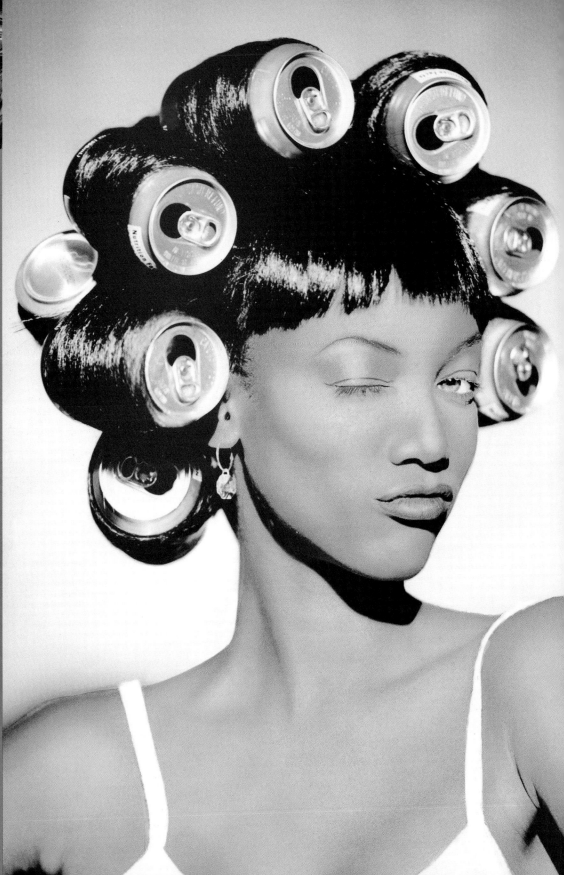

We always want
what we don't have — longer legs, higher

cheekbones, a flatter stomach, smoother skin. The same goes for our hair. Somehow the grass is always greener in somebody else's backyard. I have a friend named Kimora who has a beautiful head of naturally curly, jet black hair. But of course, she can't stand it. She says it's too pouffy, too unruly, and too uncontrollable. So, through the magic of a coloring expert and a flattening iron, she now has bone-straight, auburn hair. I have another friend Keiko, from Japan, whose hair originally was long and super straight but now is in a curly perm that mimics Kimora's natural locks.

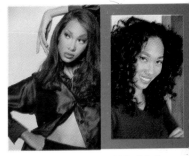

Kimora with auburn and black hair

Turning Heads

I was born with light, sandy brown hair, but I wasn't happy with it because I wanted it to look like my best friend Jamallie's hair. Hers was coal black and super shiny, and I thought it was stunning. So when I was thirteen, I went to my hairdresser and told her that my mom said it was okay to dye my hair black. Of course, that was a big fat lie. My mother was totally against my getting any permanent color until I was at least sixteen.

I thought I was **so smart...**

I took a big, floppy hat with me to the salon to wear home to cover up my dye job.

My mom didn't pay any attention when I walked in the door with it on. But when I wore it to the dinner table, it was obvious I had something to hide. I expected my mom to dramatically pull off my hat, but instead she totally ignored me. She waited until the next morning to drop the bomb.

When I woke up, she was right there in front of my face. Before I could collect my thoughts, she shouted,

"Have you lost your mind?!"

Needless to say, I was in serious trouble and was grounded for a month. But what my mother didn't realize was that I could not have cared less. I may not have been able to leave the house for thirty days, but I still had my black hair, and that was all that mattered.

It seemed so important to me back then, but today I can't even tell you why I so desperately wanted to dye my hair. Perhaps I just needed a change. Hair has that power. At the touch of a curling iron, scissors, or coloring kit, we can alter our entire look. Now that I'm a grown woman, I'm free to try out new styles and cuts in any color of the rainbow I choose, and thanks to the advice of a few professional stylists and the tricks I've picked up on my own, I now know how to use that freedom to its best advantage.

Handle with Care

There's been a lot of trial and error in my search for the perfect style. Just ask my hairdressers, Lisa Luke and Oscar James. Either one of them will tell you that my hair has weathered some serious storms: split ends, frayed edges, overprocessing, overheating, etc., etc.

My hectic schedule makes it harder for me to make those weekly appointments like I should. Fortunately, I have a hair team that's all on the same wavelength—keeping my hair healthy. Lisa, my hairdresser in Los Angeles, has known me since I was thirteen, and she makes sure that my hair is healthy and well cared for. Oscar styles my hair for most of my modeling jobs in New York, and he keeps my look updated and constantly changing.

With everything they do, that still doesn't let *me* off the hook. I have to keep reminding myself that my hair is a reflection of me, and I need to do everything I can to keep it well nourished. My stylists say it's a lesson all of us could learn. They've seen countless examples of hair damage and loss that, with some loving care, could have been avoided. Lisa has a saying:

"Hair responds to **care** but it also responds to **neglect**."

It's just like working out: **If you want to see results, you've got to put in the time.**

Getting Down to Basics

My hair is very dry and brittle and in constant need of moisture. When I don't treat it properly, it starts to break off at the ends. But now that I know how to read the signs, I can repair the damage before disaster strikes.

Having a working knowledge of our hair and its needs is critical to keeping it healthy. To come up with a hair care plan, you have to know your hair type. I've broken down the differences into three major categories:

Dry Hair Dry hair results from inadequate oil secretion from the sebaceous (oil) glands. Without the proper treatment, it can become dull, fragile, and lifeless, which leads to breakage.

Care Tips
1. Wash the hair no more than once or twice a week with a shampoo that moisturizes.
2. Condition the hair with a moisturizing conditioner.
3. Lubricate your hair with a light oil or cream hair moisturizer that locks in moisture and adds gloss. Anything heavier–like a grease containing lanolin, cocoa butter, mineral oil, or petroleum–will attract dirt, block glands, and make the hair look duller.
4. Whenever possible, go easy on heating tools like curling irons, crimping irons, and blow-dryers.
5. Avoid any styling product that contains alcohol–it has a drying effect on the hair.
6. For added shine, give yourself a once-a-month hot-oil treatment, working it into the hair and scalp.

Oily Hair Oily hair results from overproductive sebaceous glands in your scalp. A few hours after a shampoo, it often looks like it needs to be washed again.

Care Tips
1. Wash the hair with an oil-absorbing shampoo that can be used every day.
2. Use a water-based (not fatty-based) conditioner.
3. Avoid hair oils and heavy moisturizers.
4. Use light, oil-free styling products such as mousses to give added sheen and fullness.

Normal Hair Normal hair has the best of both worlds. The scalp is neither dry nor oily. The hair has good body and is manageable.

Care Tips
1. Use hair products meant for normal hair because they will neither dry it out nor overmoisturize it.
2. Think before you apply any chemical processes to the hair, such as perms, relaxers, or hair coloring; they can change normal hair into problem hair.
3. Any imbalance–too much washing or too much moisturizing–can be harmful to normal hair, so don't overdo it.

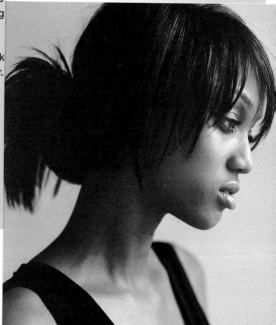

There's been an ongoing debate in the hair care industry about whether or not it's necessary to switch the kind of shampoo and conditioner you use every so often. I'm all for changing brands every few months, especially if you're not getting the same results you did when you first started using your hair care product. It's just like mopping the floors—you know how they can get that waxy buildup if you use one product for too long? Some hair care professionals believe the same thing happens to our hair. You may need to switch for a while to another product that will cut through and wear away the buildup.

As far as price is concerned, **there is no reason to believe that a product from a high-profile salon is going to work more effectively than one from the drugstore.** It's really a matter of personal preference.

WASH AND GO

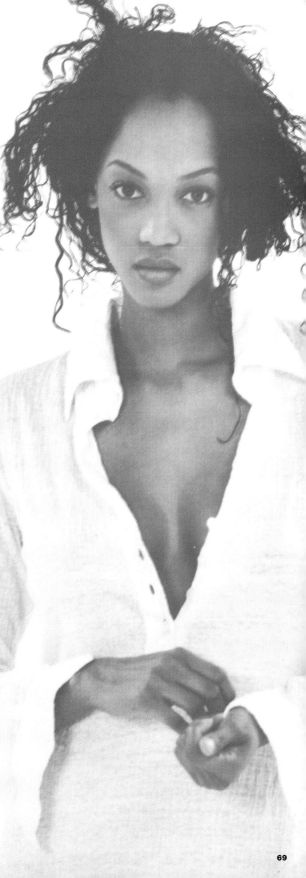

There are few things as satisfying as getting a good professional shampoo. If you've ever found yourself zoning out in the beauty salon while your hairdresser gives your hair and scalp a thorough washing and massage, you know what I mean. What I like to do when I'm at home is try to duplicate my hairdresser's technique.

I rinse my hair in lukewarm water first (anything too hot or too cold strips the hair), then I massage shampoo into my hair and scalp with the pads of my fingers (not the fingernails—they are too harsh on the scalp) until it lathers.

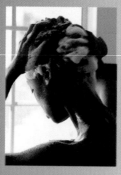

I really concentrate on stimulating the scalp because that's where the residue from too many styling products tends to linger. I rinse that out thoroughly, then repeat the entire process again. Oscar says the secret to shampooing is the water pressure; if you use pressure that's too hard, it can literally strip the nutrients right out of your hair.

The conditioning treatment is where I vary my routine. Sometimes I'll just slick my hair back with a cream hair moisturizer and call it a day. If my hair has been suffering from harsh treatment, I'll apply a penetrating protein conditioner to restore some of the moisture all those heating appliances and chemicals tend to take out. Other times, when my hair is looking a little dull, I'll give myself a hot-oil treatment that gives my hair some lubrication and shine. Whatever conditioning product I use, I make certain to distribute it evenly from roots to ends, not just on the top layer. Then I lounge around with a heating cap or shower cap on my head until the conditioner is ready to be rinsed out. I used to think that the hairdresser put a plastic cap on my head just to keep the stuff in my hair from running down my neck, but the truth is that it serves a practical purpose: The heat generated by the cap helps the conditioner to penetrate the hair shaft.

After I wash out the conditioner, I either let my hair air-dry, or I use a blow-dryer on a low setting to speed up the process.

Then I style it and *GO!*

clip tip

Don't be scissors-shy! I can't overemphasize the importance of getting regular hair trims. Keeping the ends in line prevents breakage. Otherwise, the hair starts to split up the hair shaft.

FINDING A STYLIST WHO SUITS YOU

Are you and your hair stylist in sync? I've heard at least a thousand (okay, maybe more like a hundred) war stories from people who've gone into the salon with one look in mind and come out with what the hairdresser had in mind.

I've had to confront a pushy stylist or two when they didn't want to listen to what I wanted. Once, I had someone tell me that strawberry blond streaks were "in" and if I didn't want them, then, honey, I was just gonna have to get out of his chair. I think it took me about two seconds to grab my stuff and get the heck out of there!

I haven't always been so assertive. There have been times when I've just sat there and let them have their way. I mean, you figure these people are pros and should know what they are doing, so you feel a little intimidated speaking up. But then you come out looking like a complete fool and you feel like going into hiding until the stuff grows out! And you have no one but yourself to blame.

It's very important to choose someone who knows how to work with your hair, and who can give suggestions but is comfortable doing the kind of style that you've chosen for yourself, not a cut the stylist has chosen for you.

To save you some time and aggravation, I've put together a list of things to help you find—and keep—a good stylist:

Ask around. Talk to friends, co-workers, and acquaintances about the stylists they use. My mom has no shame. She has found the greatest stylists by just walking up to someone on the street and asking, "Who does your hair? It looks so beautiful." The women are usually so flattered that they don't mind sharing the wealth.

Schedule a getting-to-know-you interview. The first appointment with a new stylist should include a consultation. This gives her an opportunity to ask you some questions about your hair care habits and any problems you may have had in the past. It also gives you a chance to find out more about her—like her specialties, the kinds of products she recommends, and, especially, her personality. Some people want a stylist who's chatty and likes to dish the dirt. If you're like me, you prefer someone who's quiet and subdued (you know, the kind who lets you read your magazine in peace). Above all, you want someone who is into hair *care* and not just hair *style* and who respects her clients' wishes.

Be realistic. Don't expect your hair stylist to work miracles. If your hair isn't long enough, curly enough, or straight enough to achieve a certain style, or is too damaged to undergo a particular process, you have to be willing to let it go. The health of your hair should take precedence over all other considerations, and chances are, your stylist can suggest a haircut that you might find just as, if not more, flattering.

Show some R-E-S-P-E-C-T. If you're going to be late or miss an appointment, you should definitely call. It's just common courtesy and will make it a whole lot easier to get an appointment the next time.

I know I'd be lost without Lisa and Oscar. Combined, I've been going to them for fourteen years, so we've built a history together. The beauty of having these relationships is that they give me honest feedback. They know when I've been neglecting my hair, and tell me so! But they're also good about giving my hair extra pampering when it needs it. Most of all, they respect my opinion, and because they do, I've continued to seek their advice on all my hair needs.

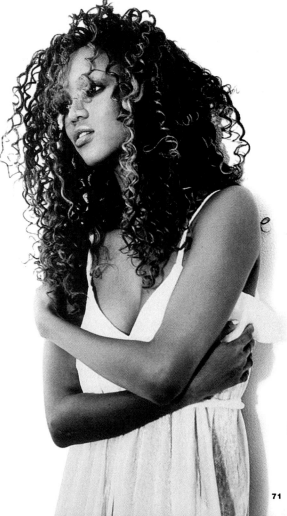

Power Tools

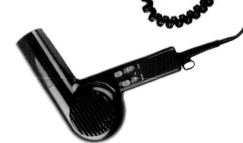

With the right styling tools, the range of looks you can achieve is wide open. Doing so many photo shoots has exposed me to just about every professional gadget you can imagine. I like to check out what tools the hair stylists use and the way they're using them because, if I admire the look they are creating, I might like to try to duplicate it at home.

So the next time you pay a visit to the hair salon, do some snooping! Take a look at the tools your stylist has on hand, and take mental notes. While the collection of blow-dryers, curlers, combs, and brushes is probably a lot more extensive and expensive than you'll need, it will give you a good idea of the kind of products you should have on hand to maintain your look.

My own list of **power tools** includes:

A wide-toothed comb made of hard rubber (metal is too rough on the hair). It's great for detangling hair when it's wet, and for longer hair it's better than combs with narrowly spaced teeth. (Hair hint: When detangling, comb hair—coated with conditioner—from the ends to the roots to prevent breakage.)

A vent brush is great for blow-drying. The best ones have widely spaced bristles with rubber-tipped ends.

A paddle brush with rounded bristles (instead of the sharp, pointed edges that can tear at your hair). Not only does it help to stimulate my scalp, but it also gives my hair a smooth finish.

A handheld blow-dryer with a cool setting. I wouldn't recommend dryers with more wattage than you need. Take a tip from a pro: Lisa uses a professional dryer and hers only reaches 1,200 watts, which she says is more than sufficient. (Hair hint: The best way to blow-dry hair is to section it into parts and dry one section at a time, keeping the dryer in a state of constant motion so that it doesn't burn the hair.)

Curling irons in several sizes. I use a small, 1/2-inch one when I want a full head of Shirley Temple–type curls; a large, 1 1/2-inch barrel for fatter, smoother curls; and a medium-size, 3/4-inch curling iron for a look that's in between.

Hot rollers with soft padding. There are some versions out now that use steam heat, which can be much kinder to the hair than the traditional dry heat. I wouldn't recommend using the old-fashioned kind with spikes–they can get tangled in the hair and cause some serious damage.

A heating cap to help conditioner penetrate the hair cuticle. Lisa wanted me to add this one to the list because too often, when we run conditioner through our hair at home, we don't leave it on long enough, so it's almost like we've never conditioned at all. Sitting with a heating cap on, even if it's for only ten minutes, makes the conditioner more effective. Most caps sell for under $20 at a beauty supply shop, which is a small investment for such a big return.

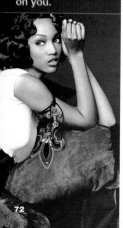

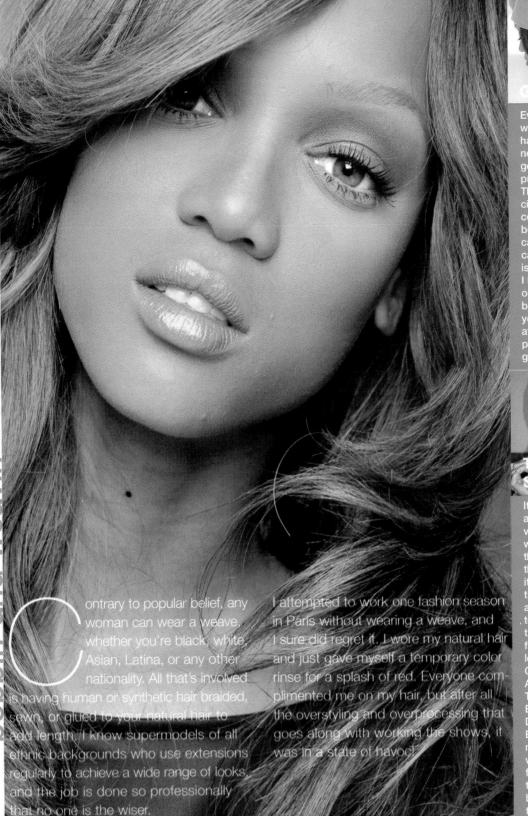

Contrary to popular belief, any woman can wear a weave, whether you're black, white, Asian, Latina, or any other nationality. All that's involved is having human or synthetic hair braided, sewn, or glued to your natural hair to add length. I know supermodels of all ethnic backgrounds who use extensions regularly to achieve a wide range of looks, and the job is done so professionally that no one is the wiser.

I attempted to work one fashion season in Paris without wearing a weave, and I sure did regret it. I wore my natural hair and just gave myself a temporary color rinse for a splash of red. Everyone complimented me on my hair, but after all the overstyling and overprocessing that goes along with working the shows, it was in a state of havoc!

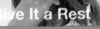

Give It a Rest

Even while we sleep, we can pamper our hair. Oscar says that no woman should go to bed without protecting her locks. That holds true especially if she sleeps on cotton pillowcases, because the cotton can be rough and cause friction, which is tough on the hair. I like to wear a silk or satin scarf to bed, but I know some of you like to look cute at night, so a satin pillowcase is also a good safeguard.

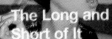

The Long and Short of It

It used to be that all we'd see on television were women with hair down to there, and we thought that was the way that it had to be. But times are a-changin' and I'm very happy to say that now that's the furthest thing from the truth! Just look at Halle Berry, Cameron Diaz, Paula Abdul, Winona Ryder, Toni Braxton, Linda Evangelista, Geena Davis, and Kim Basinger. They've all made the transition, with grace and style, from longer lengths to cropped cuts. The bottom line is that these days, anything goes!

I guess all the stress of doing five fashion shows a day for one month straight was too hard for my hair to handle. At one fashion show they wanted me to have an Afro, so they teased and crimped my hair like crazy. At my next show they wanted my hair bone-straight, so they took that crimped, teased, hair-sprayed hair and went over it with a flattening iron. At the following show they wanted dreadlocks, so the stylist twisted my hair and put beeswax in it to make it hold. And at the last stop, my hair had to look wavy and curly, so they combed the dreadlocks out and put hot curlers in for about twenty minutes. Oh, and did I mention that there's no shampooing or conditioning in between all of this? All this handiwork had my hair breaking off in clumps, so that's when I got wise to the weave.

I went to see Spice Sight, a Los Angeles stylist who specializes in hair weaves. Fortunately for me, she believes that the hair underneath the weave is just as important as the weave itself. I learned from her that with weaves, you get what you pay for. And that goes for both the quality of hair that you use and the hair stylist who performs the service. Like Spice always says, "If someone gives you a pretty nice weave, but they use cheap hair, it's a bad weave. If someone uses good-quality hair but skimps on the weaving technique, it's still a bad weave."

There are many types of hair to choose from—human, synthetic, fiber—as well as textures from stick-straight to wavy to Afro curly. My recommendation is to

go for the hair that best matches your own hair color and texture, otherwise it will be oh, so obvious that you're wearing a weave. Another important consideration in terms of style: the weaving method. There are many different techniques, each with its own pros and cons. Here are four:

1 **The braid weave.** Small braids about one inch long are made with your natural hair at the roots, then individual extension strands of hair are attached to the braids. The good thing about this method is that the extensions look almost natural. The bad thing is that your natural hair gets exposed to the same heat and chemicals that are applied to the weave, and therefore could be damaged.

2 **The sew-in weave.** Here the extensions are literally sewn to your natural hair with a needle and thread. If secured too tightly, the threads can tug at your natural hair, get tangled, and pull it out.

3 **The bond weave.** It sounds exactly like what it is. Extensions are bonded to your natural hair with a substance that works like glue. Many stylists like to use this one because it is quick and easy to execute—we're talking twenty minutes in many cases. Unfortunately, its shelf life is just as long. The weave loosens up after only a few shampoos. In addition, when you go to have the extensions removed, the bonding material usually leaves a glue residue. If you don't get all of the residue out and try to comb through your hair, it can cause considerable damage.

4 **The tree weave.** This one is my personal favorite because it allows for complete protection of my natural hair. First the natural hair is braided into cornrows and, as Spice braids, she adds extensions to the cornrows. This way,

the hair isn't exposed to any kind of heat. This kind of weave can last for up to two and a half months.

Once a stylist has carefully added the extensions, trimmed it, curled it, styled it, and sent you on your way, it's time for you to take over. Spice suggests a nighttime regimen of scalp massage, followed by wrapping, braiding, or pinning the hair up into a bun to keep it from tangling overnight.

The ironic thing about weaves is that you could be adding on hair but losing your own if you don't take care of it, which is why I don't leave extensions in my hair for long. You may be proud of your new look, but when that weave comes out, you want to be proud of what's underneath and naturally yours. After years of careful attention, my hair is in such good shape now that I no longer need to wear a weave. But if you see any photos of me with hair down to my butt, just know that it ain't my natural hair.

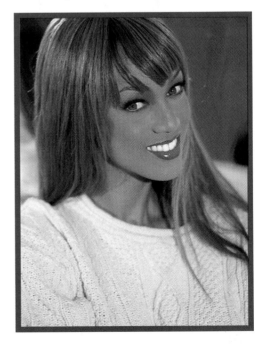

TWISTED SISTERS

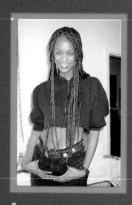

I've had my hair braided many ways over the years: cornrows, dooky braids, French, and twists: I love having braids because I can just wake up in the mornings and not worry about what to do with my hair.

I remember the first time I got dooky braids (big, thick braids). Being the penny-pincher I am, I was excited that I had found someone who charged me only $35 for labor and $15 for the bags of hair to be added for thickness and length. I sat in the braider's chair for about an hour while she tugged and pulled and twisted my hair and the extensions into long, two-tone colored braids. At one point, she tugged a little too hard and I told her I thought it was too tight. She replied, "Girl, sit still. I've got to do it this way so your braids will last." She said she didn't want them unraveling five minutes after I left her chair. So I patiently sat through the discomfort until she finished.

When she swiveled the chair around to face the mirror and I saw how they looked, man oh man did I think I was just too cute. That day I drove to all of my friends' houses to show off my new Nubian tresses. But when I got home that evening, my pleasure turned to pain. My head was hurting so badly that I wanted to run and scream. It hurt to talk, it hurt to eat, and I couldn't even think about smiling because the pain was too intense.

Anyway, I ended up taking those braids out of my head then and there. After I let my scalp recover for a week, I went to another braider, P.J., and had her re-do them, but these were looser. This time around, I was looking good—and feeling good too.

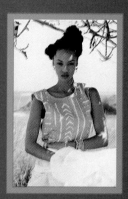

Here are a few things to watch out for if you wear or are thinking about getting braids:

1. Be sure the braids are not too tight. You will have to get them re-done more frequently, but you'll be more comfortable.

2. Pay attention to your hairline. Braids that are too tight around this area will cause your "edges" to break off and can create permanent hair loss over time.

3. Don't leave braids in too long. This will cause your hair to mat around the braids, making it difficult to remove them, and could lead to hair loss.

4. Oil or moisturize the scalp. It relieves dryness and irritation caused by the braids.

5. Wash hair and scalp once a week with shampoo and a conditioner. Many women feel washing will make braids come apart, but a clean scalp is a healthy scalp. Using witch hazel on the scalp once a week and washing hair every other week is another way to keep the scalp clean.

6. When you remove your braids, wait at least a week before putting in new ones. It allows your hair and scalp to rest from all the tension.

Some people are under the impression that having braids limits the number of hair styles you can wear, but that's not true. Just look at singer/actress Brandy. You rarely see her with the same hairdo. She's worn her braids in every possible way imaginable, from upsweep 'dos to curly ringlets, from auburn-colored plaits to jet black minibraids so long they grazed her backside.

Advice for DYE-HARDS

Based on my earlier experience with hair color (remember, the dye job that got me grounded?) you might think I would be a big fan, but I'm not, and with good reason. A few months after I first started modeling, I decided to have my hair dyed. Only instead of going to my regular hairdresser, I decided to try someone new. Big mistake! I asked him to dye my hair a shade lighter. But the color came out too light—we're talking platinum blond! Then to fix it, he tried to darken my hair and the color came out almost black.

All that chemical processing was too much for my hair to take, and it broke off, to the point where I had to wear wigs. It was either that or walking around half bald! And since I didn't want to join the Hair Club for Men, I had no choice but to put a wig on my head. Normally my hair grows back quickly, but because of this abuse, it didn't recover for months.

Ever since that incident, I have been extremely careful with color. But that doesn't mean I shy away from it—I just stick to what I know my hair can handle, a guideline I think everyone should keep in mind.

If you're looking to make a dramatic color change, I think it's safest to put your hair in the hands of professional colorists, because they know best how to protect your hair during the process.

If you want to change your color slightly or just add a few highlights, then an at-home color kit should do. (It's also a lot less pricey than what you'd spend in a salon.) My advice is to read, read, read the packaging before you plunk down your dollars. I asked a few of my hairdresser friends to help me sift through some colorist lingo:

If the box says:	It means:
Temporary color	Product has no ammonia or peroxide.
	The color does not penetrate the hair shaft.
	The color will tint, not lighten or darken, the hair.
	The color will fade after a couple of shampoos.
Semipermanent color	Product contains low levels of peroxide.
	The color will penetrate the hair shaft.
	The color lasts up to two months, but eventually fades.
Permanent color	Product strips pigment from the hair and deposits a new color.
	Process is harder on the hair and not recommended for relaxed or damaged hair.
	New growth at the roots will stand out once the dyed hair starts to grow out.

Every time I walk into a drugstore, I can't believe the number of hair coloring products on the shelves. You name it, they've got it: kits for streaks, soft highlights, all over color, changing from light to dark and back again. For the most part, these at-home hair enhancers are safe and nondamaging, just as long as you follow the directions precisely.

Choosing a Color
Adding color doesn't have to be drastic. In fact, I prefer shades that bring out my hair's natural honey brown undertones.

The worst way to pick a color is by the picture on the package. The photograph could have been retouched, or the way the model's hair takes color might be totally different from yours. Sometimes there's a color chart on the back of some boxes, and that is a better indicator because it gives you an idea of what kind of shade you'll end up with based on the color you already have.

You can also take the plunge and purchase the color, but test it out first on a small section of your hair. If the strand test suits you, you can proceed with confidence.

After-Color Care
Color-treated hair requires extra care. To maintain the color and keep your hair healthy, I recommend using shampoos and conditioners made especially for color-treated hair. Not only do they have penetrating moisturizers built in to keep hair from drying out, but they also help hair hold on to color so that it doesn't fade as quickly.

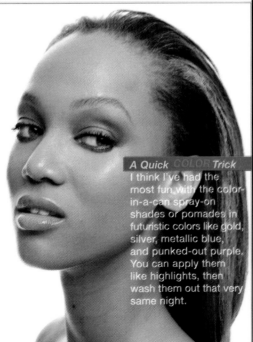

A Quick COLOR Trick
I think I've had the most fun with the color-in-a-can spray-on shades or pomades in futuristic colors like gold, silver, metallic blue, and punked-out purple. You can apply them like highlights, then wash them out that very same night.

Dreaded Dandruff
Those white flakes and annoying itch could mean that your scalp is either producing too much oil or getting too little. Or your body might be going through a dry spell (this is especially true in winter, but can also occur when you don't drink enough water). In any case, the scalp cells start to shed in clumps that cling to your hair, scalp, and sometimes your clothes.

The problem is easily addressed by washing your hair and scalp with an antidandruff shampoo at least once a week. This will not only keep the hair and scalp clean but will prevent product buildup. Sulfur shampoos are a good solution for oily scalps because they slow down oil production. Milder antidandruff shampoos work best for dry scalps because they don't sap the scalp of any moisture. Never use dandruff shampoos as a substitute for your regular shampoo because they contain chemicals that can be harsh on hair if used for prolonged periods. They're just a stand-in until the condition goes away. With more serious cases—severe itching and flaking, a reddened scalp—you might want to consult a doctor who can direct you to the right prescription products.

One side note: In some cases, the flaking you see isn't dandruff at all, but the result of using too many hair products, such as pomades, heavy hair greases, and setting gels, that contain alcohol. Even in these cases, simply give the hair and scalp a good cleansing.

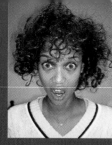

Everyone has those horror hair days when the curling iron just doesn't seem to be acting right, or one side of your hair looks better than the other so you try to fix the problem with some hair spray and your hair goes super stiff, so you layer on the conditioning gel to soften it up a bit, but that just makes it look pasty, and now the only way you can fix it is to wash your hair and start from scratch, which you don't have time to do.

Whenever I'm going through a bad-hair day, I slick my hair back with some cream hair moisturizer or pomade and pull it into a ponytail or a bun. Women with short hair can also try the slick trick by adding a side part and smoothing down the hair with gel. If your hair is curly and you want to take a walk on the wild side, you can add water and conditioner to the hair, scrunch it with your hands, and let it air dry. If things are REALLY bad, a hat will usually do.

STRICTLY for the PROS

Sometimes when our hair is in need of some serious repair, we try to fix it ourselves instead of seeking help from a professional. Bad move! Most of the time, we just end up making it worse. Here are a few cases when a pro is definitely the way to go:

CONDITION: **Fried and Frizzed**
(Bad Relaxer or Curly Perm)

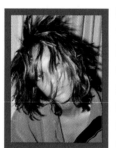

CAUSES: Leaving the chemicals in too long until the hair is either bone-straight (in the case of a relaxer) or so curly it frizzes up (in the case of a curly permanent), or applying chemicals to hair that's already permed or relaxed instead of only to the new growth. The latter usually happens with do-it-yourself jobs, but can sometimes happen at the hands of a professional.

My mom has experienced that horror. Not too long ago, she went to a new hairdresser to have a relaxer put in her hair, with disastrous results. It was one of those places where one person puts the relaxer in, another person washes it out, and another person styles it. Unfortunately, the person who was supposed to wash the relaxer out was preoccupied with something else and wasn't paying attention, so the chemicals started to burn my mom's scalp. By the time it was all over, her scalp was chemically burned.

A few days later, scabs formed which, over time, left permanent scars on her scalp. Her hair broke off, and from that point on, she had to give up relaxers altogether. But with the help of Lisa Luke, she now has a beautiful head of hair again.

CURE: A hair care specialist can assess the damage, and make recommendations accordingly. Depending on the degree of damage, sometimes hair can be conditioned back into shape. If the hair is overprocessed beyond repair, there isn't much a stylist can do to bring it back. At that point, you will have to have the overprocessed hair cut off. But don't panic! A good hairdresser will style the hair in a way that flatters and camouflages the problem. Just know that restoring your hair to its natural, healthy state will definitely take more than one visit.

CONDITION: **Bad Breaks**
(Split Ends)

CAUSES: Overusing styling tools–blow-drying on high settings, combing and brushing the hair too roughly–and not getting timely trims are the biggest culprits.

CURE: Going in for a good trim is the BEST way to combat this problem. It's important to address the problem early on. The longer you wait, the greater the chance that the split will move up the hair shaft and do more harm.

CONDITION: Disappearing Acts
(Thinning Hairline/Hair Loss)

CAUSES: Constantly cinching the hair into a ponytail, braiding the hair too tightly at the edges—even stress can take its toll. Hair accessories such as hats and rubber bands worn too often, poor eating habits, and some prescription medications can also lead to hair loss.

CURE: First and foremost, be sure that your diet is well-balanced. Hair loss is often a sign that the body is not getting enough nutrients, such as iron and vitamins A and E.

If diet isn't the problem, consider how you have been treating your hair and change any damaging habits (like the ones mentioned earlier) that could be causing the thinning.

Many salons have staff members, trained in trichology (the scientific study of hair), whose job it is to keep the hair and scalp healthy. One of these "hair medics" should be able to diagnose the problem and recommend the right course of action, which could mean anything from a change in the products you use to a change of hairstyle that will give your hair a rest.

If the problem is beyond the salon's scope of knowledge, and the hair loss is excessive, then it's time to consult a dermatologist who typically can diagnose the problem and recommend the proper treatment.

CONDITION: Color Catastrophe
(Bad Dye Job)

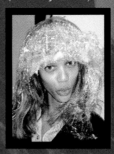

CAUSES: Leaving the product in too long; mixing different colors/kits that don't belong together to achieve a certain color; making a drastic color change (for example, from dark brunette to platinum blond).

CURE: This situation usually leaves the hair in a weakened state that requires pampering by a professional hair colorist, because not every stylist is an expert with color. He or she will most likely start by reconditioning the hair before any further corrective measures are taken. It may also be necessary to trim off the ends damaged by the coloring so that you can make a fresh start.

Sometimes no matter how much effort you put into your 'do, there are days when the 'fro frizzes up, the locks go limp, the weave looks like a wig, and the style gives you nothing but static. Through many trials, and lots of error, I've learned the hard way.

Our hair is a reflection of ourselves, an expression of our individuality. So have fun. Whatever shape your tresses take, remember that it's your hair and your choice.

The key is keeping it healthy and strong.

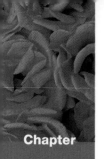

My grandparents are from Louisiana and Texas—two states where good cookin' is in the genes—so the kitchen was always humming at our house. Everywhere I turned there were mouth-watering foods in abundance—fried chicken wings, barbecue ribs, macaroni and cheese, honeyed ham, smothered pork chops, and candied yams. Holidays were the best. My grandma Marie used to have ten different kinds of desserts, from triple-layered German chocolate cake to deep-dish sweet potato pies, lined up at Christmas. And my great-grandmother Fannie used to make mashed potatoes with more cream and butter than potatoes.

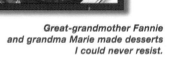

Great-grandmother Fannie and grandma Marie made desserts I could never resist.

I was taught to enjoy food, not fear it.

To this day, my family never celebrates without some kind of grubbing being involved. Whenever something groundbreaking or spectacular happens in my career, my mom and I treat ourselves to dinner at a fancy-schmancy restaurant and just pig out.

But I'll admit that I've also turned to food in bad times.

When I first started modeling and was living in Paris, I was so lonely and homesick that I made a list of every McDonald's, Häagen-Dazs, and Burger King in the city, and I'd eat at one of them every single day.

I have made
a commitment to myself
to eat to live,
not live to eat
and to stay active.

And so far,
I'm sticking to it
...........**kind of.**

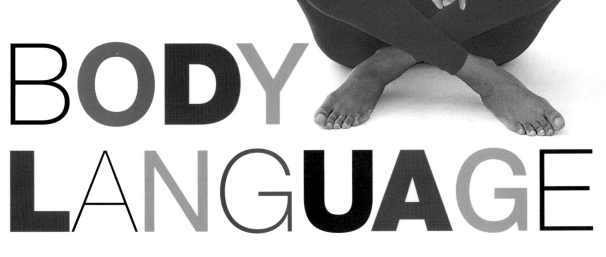

BODY LANGUAGE

There Must Be Something in the Water

Whenever I'm thirsty, the first thing I reach for is lemonade, iced tea, or some type of carbonated drink. I just love the taste of sweetened liquids, especially with meals.

I was raised on Kool-Aid. My brother and I were in charge of making it, and we used to argue about which flavor to use. I liked cherry and he preferred grape. But one thing we didn't argue about was how much sugar to put in —at least ten scoops! It was absolutely ridiculous, but I guess that desire for sugared beverages has never left me.

I know my water intake is low. I simply don't like the taste—or lack of it. But when I go for a long time without drinking pure H_2O, I notice the effects immediately. My skin gets all dry and flaky, and starts to break out. And after I take a little tinkle, I check out the contents of the toilet and that pee looks a little more yellow than it should.

Water flushes out the toxic waste in our system and keeps the body functioning efficiently. If your water intake is low, those toxins will hang around and start causing all kinds of trouble. Water also keeps the body from dehydrating by replenishing the fluids we lose when we work up a sweat. So gulp down at least eight glasses a day. Then check out that toilet—the water will be so clear it'll almost look like you never used it.

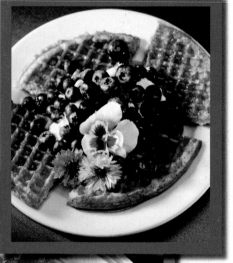

I missed the food back home so much that I even had my mom send me huge care packages of junk food. She thought I was just periodically snacking on these treats, but I was eating sandwich cookies for breakfast, peanut brittle for lunch, and caramel corn for dinner. At one point during a fashion show I almost fainted on the runway because of my poor nutrition.

So I guess you could say that food has been a fundamental part of my existence. But as I've gotten older, I've decided that I don't want food to rule my life. So I've made some adjustments, not just in my eating habits, but in my total approach to health.

I don't starve and I don't deprive myself. I eat some of everything I like, but maybe just not as much of it as I'd like to. That, combined with regular exercise, keeps me in pretty good shape. I have made a commitment to myself to eat to live, not to live to eat, and to stay active. And so far, I'm sticking to it........kind of.

Food Attitudes

Because I model for a living, people either expect me to be extremely particular about what I eat, or in many cases, to eat hardly at all. They are so surprised when they find out not only that I like to eat, but that I'm not shy about it. I dig right in! I can't tell you the number of modeling trips I've been on where I have been dining with the crew and caused a commotion because I had a full breakfast. There was this one time when I was eating bacon, eggs, and waffles with extra syrup and butter, while the other people ordered juice and an apple. From the strange looks I'd get, I knew people were thinking, "How can she eat like that and stay in shape?"

Of course Clayton, my trainer, would much rather I eat something sensible. He eats oatmeal with no milk or sugar (Yuck!), and encourages me to eat a low-fat breakfast too. Many fitness experts say that if you must pig out, breakfast is the best meal for it, because then you'll have the rest of the day to burn it off. There are also the energy benefits. I know I can't function on an empty stomach, so I make sure that I feed my body enough fuel to get me through the day. But, of course, it has to be the right kind of fuel. And I know that eating bacon, eggs, and waffles with extra syrup and butter every day ain't the right fuel. And that's something I just have to deal with.

My family's obsession with southern food makes it even harder to eat healthy. Whenever I go to a relative's house, they say, "Girl, you are so skinny, somebody fix her a plate." The only problem is that most of those foods are high in fat, salt, sugar, and cholesterol. Consumed in large portions over long periods of time, this kind of eating can contribute to all kinds of illnesses, from high blood pressure to various heart problems. In my family, we have a history of diabetes, strokes, and heart disease. My grandmother's sister died of hypertension. My mom's dad was diabetic. My mom has a constant weight struggle, which puts her at risk for these family illnesses.

I worry about her succumbing to the same diseases that have been in our family for generations.

So I'm trying to set an example for her. It's important that I pay attention to what I'm putting into my body, because genetically I'm prone to be a victim of these diseases.

I admit, though, that eating right isn't always easy, and sometimes I slip up. But the way I deal with it is by bargaining with myself. I'll allow myself to eat some buffalo wings today, as long as I double up on the healthy foods and cut back on fat tomorrow. The hardest part is keeping on track, and I constantly slip up. But I'm beginning to realize that if I take it slow and accept that it's impossible to change my eating habits overnight, I'm more likely to stick with the program.

COW JUICE

One new diet craze is to eliminate dairy products from your diet entirely. And yes, you might lose weight, but your bones will pay for it. Have you ever wondered why so many elderly women have such poor posture? Most likely, those stooped shoulders and backs are symptoms of osteoporosis, a loss of bone mass or density that leads to fractures. Women are particularly vulnerable to the disease, because we start out with less bone density than men do. If we don't eat properly and monitor our calcium intake, the problem worsens. Smoking, caffeine, excessive alcohol, and insufficient exercise make us even more susceptible. The earlier we introduce calcium into our diets—milk, cheese, yogurt— the better off we'll be.

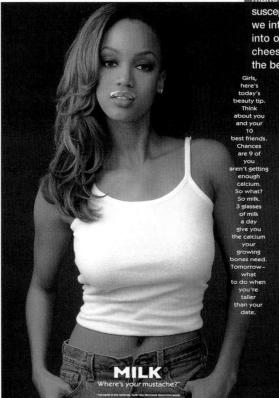

Girls, here's today's beauty tip. Think about you and your 10 best friends. Chances are 9 of you aren't getting enough calcium. So what? So milk. 3 glasses of milk a day give you the calcium your growing bones need. Tomorrow— what to do when you're taller than your date.

MILK
Where's your mustache?

Body LOVE

I f there's one period in my life that I don't ever wish to relive, it's puberty. The awkward stage started when I was eleven years old. Over about a three-month time span, I lost nearly twenty pounds and grew three inches. Of course, the growth spurt made me tower over everyone in my class, including the teacher! I was five feet, nine inches tall, as thin as a rail, and miserable. I was so skinny

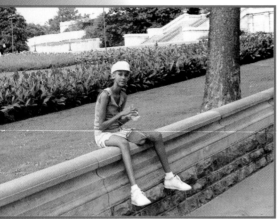

that even my teachers began to worry. They all thought I had an eating disorder. My mother took me to the best doctors to try to find out if I had a medical problem, but after poking me with needles and monitoring me on machines, they unanimously agreed that I was in perfect health and that there was absolutely nothing to worry about. They all said that one day I would just start gaining weight.

But of course that was easier said than done. Before my body went through all these bizarre physical changes, I was extroverted, had a lot of friends, and was always in trouble for trying to show off and be the class clown. But when I lost the weight and grew so tall, I became self-conscious and introverted. I rarely showed my face in public, and when I did, it was buried in a book. I'd do anything to avoid the rude stares from people, and I'd try to block out the things they

would say, like, "Gosh, she's so skinny she'd blow over if a big wind came along," and, "Quick, somebody give her a pork chop." Most of the time I stayed locked up in my room.

I felt so uncomfortable in such a skinny body, and did some pretty unhealthy things to attempt to gain the weight back, including stuffing myself with artery-clogging, fattening foods. I tried to eat as many fried things as possible and I'd make myself chocolate-and-peanut butter ice cream shakes every night before bedtime. But nothing seemed to work. I'd get on the scale every day, but my weight stayed the same. Ninety-eight pounds.

As I moved into my teens and all the popular girls at my school started to develop breasts and hips, my body just stayed the same—straight and narrow. I don't think I felt good about my figure until I turned seventeen, when I began to gain weight and actually started developing some curves. Ironically, this is around the same time my modeling career began to take off.

Just when I started loving my body, I had to deal with an entirely new set of worries. Even though people were hiring me, curves and all, I soon became self-conscious. I wear a size eight, but compared to some of the other less-endowed models in the industry, I'm full-figured. Early in my career, my size made it hard to work with some designers, because their clothing was tailored with a

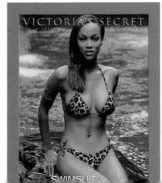

size-two or -four model in mind. Their attitude was that if you wanted to work for them, you had to be able to fit into their clothes—no ifs, ands, or buts. And since that wasn't my size, I'd lose out on some major jobs.

Iman

Claudia Schiffer

Thankfully, there were some role models in the business I could look to, such as Iman, Helena Christiansen, Claudia Schiffer, and Cindy Crawford, whose shapely physiques proved that you didn't have to be bone-thin to be successful. Looking at them made me stop listening to those people who tried to make me feel insecure because of my size, and I began to appreciate my body for what it was.

Reading my fan mail makes me appreciate my body type even more. To someone on the street, I may look pretty slim, but in the modeling world, my curves are the exception, not the rule. People tell me that they are pleased that I am not super skinny and that I've "got some meat on my bones." Those thousands of positive letters helped me realize how important it is for women to be able to open up a magazine and see a variety of models with varying shapes and body types.

I've spent a lot of time worrying about my body type, tripping on insecurities and doubting myself. But I decided that I'm not going to obsess over things I can't do anything about. When I look in the mirror, I see that I have curvy hips and full breasts and that they're really not going anywhere. But that's okay. They're where they were meant to be.

I've spent a lot of time worrying about my body type, tripping on insecurities and doubting myself.

The Food BLUES

We all hear stories about models going to an extreme to lose or maintain their weight. And I wish I could say that eating disorders haven't infiltrated the modeling industry, but I have to admit that that's simply not the case. I met a young model a few years ago who really had me worried. She didn't feel good about her body and told me that she didn't want to have hips and breasts. She would call her developing breasts fat, and bind them with gauze for a flat-chested appearance. She said the new waif look was in, and she was losing out on jobs because of her curves. She later proceeded to eat less and less, until she fainted. Thankfully, her family recognized the problem and got her some help.

There was another model Ma and I saw backstage in Paris at one of the fashion shows who had a similar problem. My mom, who hadn't seen her in a while, was shocked to see how thin she was. She said, "Honey, you've lost *so* much weight. You look like you've lost twenty pounds or something. You don't look well." And the model replied, "Really? Thank you!" My mom was trying to tell her that she looked sickly, but all she heard was that she looked skinny and took my mom's concern as a compliment.

People always blame models for the rise of eating disorders, and yes, the industry does have something to do with the phenomenon because so many of us are extremely thin. But I believe the slim images that television constantly bombards us with, from our favorite sitcom stars to the weight-conscious women in cereal commercials, is a much more powerful influence than any high-fashion magazine could ever be. More little girls watch TV than read magazines.

What's funny is that if we turned back the page a few hundred years, we would see that the concept of the ideal body changed with the times. At one time, round, full-figured women like those who modeled for Rubens's nude paintings were considered the height of sensuality, while skinny women were shunned. But that look eventually went out of fashion, replaced by 1920s flapper styles that encouraged women to bind their breasts to appear flat-chested. In the 1950s, voluptuous sex symbols like Marilyn Monroe were the epitome of femininity and beauty. I don't know if her size fourteen to sixteen figure would receive the same overwhelming approval today. The 1960s brought an early wave of waifs; pencil-thin models like Twiggy ruled the runways. By the 1980s, athletic bodies were considered the new ideal, but that has given way in the 1990s to an emphasis on lean and mean, where there's no such thing as too skinny.

Men, on the other hand, rarely go through these changes. For the most part, a toned body is their main goal, no matter what. Throughout the decades, from Steve Reeves to Arnold Schwarzenegger, from Kirk Douglas to Sylvester Stallone, from Burt Lancaster to Jean-Claude Van Damme, from Yul Brynner to Jackie Chan, from Paul Robeson to Wesley Snipes, from Tarzan to Superman to Batman, they all have the same strong, athletic builds. But with women, it's an entirely different

THERE IS NO **ONE** BODY IMAGE THAT SUITS EVERY- ONE.

thing. We'd probably save ourselves a lot of anxiety if we followed their example. But that's easier said than done.

Once we get past the basic idea that women should be healthy and fit, there is no one body image that suits everyone. We are all individuals, coming from different places in our lives. I was once interviewed for an article on the difference between how white and black women viewed their bodies, and it was very revealing. The white

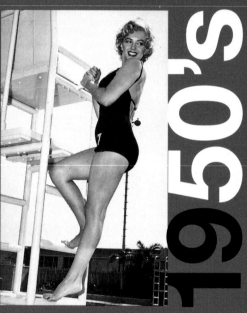

women tended to aspire to model-thin proportions, whereas with the black women, it was the complete opposite. I wasn't surprised with the finding that in the black community, it was more acceptable to have broader hips and thicker thighs. To the black women, being skinny would make them the subject of ridicule.

I guess that's another reason why I felt so uncomfortable in my own body. Whenever I was around my white friends at school, they admired my slimness, but when I would go home to my black family and friends, they would tease me about needing to put on some pounds. My younger cousin had similar issues with body image. At home and at school, she would spend hours in the bathroom, but no one understood why until one day my aunt was called to school for a conference. There she found out that my little cousin had been stuffing her hips and padding her backside with toilet tissue to make it look like she had more goin' on than she really did.

1960's

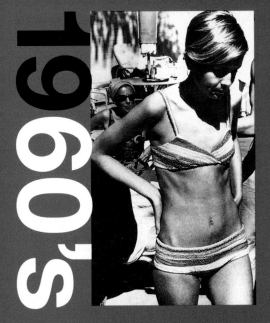

What my cousin and I have since come to realize is that a strong body image is all about how you see yourself. Once you accept you for you, nothing anyone else says makes a difference. Some people, however, can't seem to get past the scrutiny. Instead of laughing it off, they turn it inward, obsessing over their bodies, sometimes with dangerous consequences. Eating disorders such as anorexia nervosa and bulimia, which I will elaborate on later, are some of the worst-case scenarios. Doctors believe that many cases of eating disorders begin

as control issues. Some women try to take strict control of their bodies because they feel it's the only thing they can have complete control over.

I guess they're reacting to what they see in our society. All we have to do is look around us to see that if you're thin, you're in. Images in the media teach us that thin people are energetic, perfect, happy, and loved, while overweight people are lazy, unhappy, dateless, and loveless. Weight-loss commercials and print ads have women believing that if they can achieve thinness, then all their troubles will be over.

The only thing that truly makes us feel good about our bodies is accepting them for what they are, and working with what we have. Here are some places to start:

Praise your strong points, both inside and out. Everyone has something about themselves worth applauding, and it doesn't have to be something physical. Good grades, good friends, and a good attitude are excellent reasons to be proud of yourself.

Don't believe the hype. Remember early on when I talked about how photographers retouch photographs? Most of the time that means they've taken out all the cellulite and extra flesh, so that the picture you're seeing isn't based on reality. So don't worry about what the media says is "in" or "out" in terms of body types. Just concentrate on making your body as healthy and strong as it can be.

Talk it out. Sometimes sharing our feelings of insecurity and uncertainty with someone who is willing to listen and won't judge us can make us feel ten times better.

THE ONLY THING THAT TRULY MAKES US FEEL GOOD ABOUT OUR BODIES IS ACCEPTING THEM FOR WHAT THEY ARE.

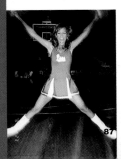

FOOD IS NOT OPTIONAL: We need it to survive. Yet when a woman views food as an enemy, she may resort to extreme—and sometimes life-threatening—measures to stay thin. A distorted body image can lead to debilitating eating disorders. In many cases, seeking help from a support group or health care professional is the only way to break the cycle.

ANOREXIA NERVOSA	BULIMIA	COMPULSIVE EXERCISING
What it is: An eating disorder in which sufferers starve themselves to become thinner. The signs: Dramatic weight loss, depression, obsession with being thin, overwhelming fear of gaining weight. Starts with occasional diets and worsens with age. Some cases can last for five to ten years. The effects: Wild mood swings, light-headed feeling, menstrual flow stops, and lanugo (a ducklinglike fur the body produces to keep warm, a natural reaction to weight loss).	What it is: An eating disorder in which sufferers go on eating binges, then force themselves to throw up or use laxatives to eliminate the food from their bodies. The signs: Eating excessively, then running to the bathroom to vomit after meals; frequent fasting; dramatic weight changes; chronic bad breath. The effects: Mood swings, depression, burning of the lining of the esophagus and the digestive tract, and tooth decay caused by stomach acids.	What it is: A disorder in which sufferers are obsessed with exercising. The signs: Must exercise after every meal to prevent weight gain; work out to get thin, not to maintain health; exercise too often or too strenuously. The effects: Miss out on other things because too busy exercising, get cranky and nervous when can't exercise, constant exhaustion from overexertion.

DISORDERS DEMYSTIFIED

People mainly put the emphasis on two eating disorders—anorexia nervosa and bulimia. But there are others that don't get this amount of media attention and can be very serious.

Eating Disorder:	What to watch for:
Night-eating syndrome	Eats about 50 percent of meals during the night. Will wake up hungry and eat a series of small meals in the middle of the night, but will skip breakfast. Leads to irregular eating habits. Disturbs sleep rhythms.
Binge-eating disorder	Frequent bingeing followed by massive guilt. Portions are excessive (for example, an entire gallon of ice cream). Usually accompanied by bouts of depression.
Restricted eating	Excessive dieting rituals, such as strict calorie counting. Skip meals, even when experiencing hunger pangs. Occasionally will blow the diet and indulge, then feel guilty and go back to an even more restricted diet.

Battling Obesity

Let's face reality: We live in a thin-obsessed world. So for the overweight and obese, life can be harsh. Obesity can be caused by any number of factors, including heredity, a medical condition, overeating, and not getting enough exercise. Some obese people may eat to distract themselves from their problems, which temporarily dissolves the pain, but after the food is consumed, it only causes guilt, which leads to more stress and emotional upset and then more eating. It's a vicious cycle. Over time, obesity can also lead to serious health problems, such as heart disease and strokes.

Getting healthy starts with a doctor's visit to develop a sensible eating program. Some people might find support groups such as Overeaters Anonymous or Weight Watchers to be helpful. If you decide to participate in a weight-loss plan, be realistic. The people in those commercials did lose weight, but it took time and patience. And you have no idea what they look like now. Once they've completed the program and returned to the real world, facing real food and not the program's diet shakes or prepackaged meals, have they gained all the weight back?

Losing weight is not easy. You'll have good and bad days, and you are not a failure if you backslide occasionally. The key is having the strength to get back on track. Just remember to keep your eyes on your goal— **to be healthy.**

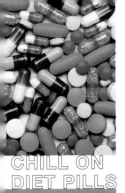

Working It Out

I've known about the importance of exercise from the time I was seven. My mother was an excellent fitness role model for me. She used to organize a group of her friends to come over to our house and have exercise classes. At the time, Jane Fonda's workout videos were extremely popular, so my mom would just pop one in and they'd begin.

She was the perfect one to lead the group because she showed no mercy. While the rest of the class was yelling, "Oh, Carolyn, stop it, I'm dying!" she'd say, "No way, honey, keep on going!" She could do nonstop sit-ups while keeping count aloud for the rest of the class to follow. And back then, my mamma had a figure on her that could put Demi Moore to shame. She was living proof that if I stuck to something, the payoff would be tremendous.

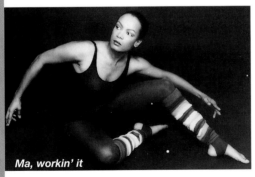

Ma, workin' it

When I first started getting into a regular exercise routine, looking buff was my primary motivation. Wanting to be healthy and fit had absolutely nothing to do with it. I saw Janet Jackson in her "If" video, and said, "Damn, I want my body to look just like that!"

I would work out in the gym for a couple of weeks and every day I would run home and strip down naked in front of the mirror, hoping to see Janet's abs staring back at me. But all I'd see was Tyra's same old stomach. And since I didn't see any new bulging muscles, I'd say to myself, "What's the point? It's not worth it," and I'd give up on my exercise plan.

When I look back now, I realize how unrealistic my goals were. I was never really happy with working out because I didn't see immediate results. I think part of it was also that I was bored with the gym—treadmills, StairMasters, buff guys walking around in skimpy unitards. I didn't find it exciting at all, and dragging myself there was sheer agony.

I think a lot of people have similar problems with exercise—they forget that it can be a lot of fun. Once I began to expand my ideas of what exercising could involve, I started looking forward to getting my lazy butt out of that bed and doing something that was physically active every day.

I prefer to work out early in the day, when there are few people out and the streets are peaceful. The slight chill of the morning air energizes me. I feel the sun warm my back, breathe in the fragrance of grass, flowers, the ocean, and listen to nothing but my own thoughts—it's like a little slice of heaven.

Because I enjoy natural scenery, when I'm at home in sunny Los Angeles, I prefer outdoor training. Running—which is a great cardiovascular workout as well as a great leg toner—is my favorite. I try not to make it too monotonous, because I'll easily become bored, so I switch it around a bit. (I also make sure I wear a sports bra with any exercise routine for added support. It prevents premature drooping.)

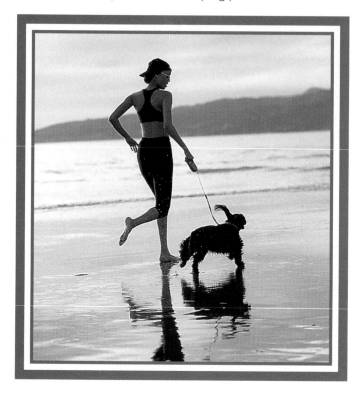

Running with Midnight on Santa Monica Beach

Sometimes I do a three-mile run along the beach. Sand is obviously much softer than a paved track, so you really have to dig in your heels, but I like it because it forces my muscles to work harder. I also like running in the park. Grass is a natural cushion against injury because it absorbs the pressure you're putting on your feet, ankles, and knees. Now that I think about it, there aren't too many places where I won't run. I used to run through a shopping mall with a friend, but we had to stop that because mall security thought we were shoplifting. My biggest fitness accomplishment yet has been completing a 10K run (6.2 miles) without walking. Now it's routine for me to run 10K races.

When I want to vary my routine, I run up and down stairs. There are outdoor stairs all over Los Angeles that athletic people like to use in their workouts. I prefer wooden stairs because they are softer and easier on the joints. When I'm a little tired, I do about three sets of stairs—two hundred steps each—up and down, with my friends. When I'm working up to my fullest potential, I push myself to do six complete cycles.

I can't tell you how much of a difference working out has made in my overall outlook. The most noticeable improvement has been in my stamina. Once I get that blood pumping, I have incredible energy that lasts throughout the rest of the day.

The benefits have spilled over into my work. When I'm working out, I actually pose with more confidence. I don't worry as much as I used to about how my stomach, thighs, or butt are going to look when I turn to the side, thinking that there's going to be something wiggling or jiggling. Even if that's the case, it doesn't matter because I have such a positive mind-set after exercising that I don't obsess as much.

And most of all, my attitude has changed. When I look in the mirror now, I'm not looking for bulging muscles. I just admire my progress. I still have a ways to go, but I'm not in any rush. I've learned to work within my own pace. When I see how far I've come, I know that my persistence is paying off, and that makes me feel darn good.

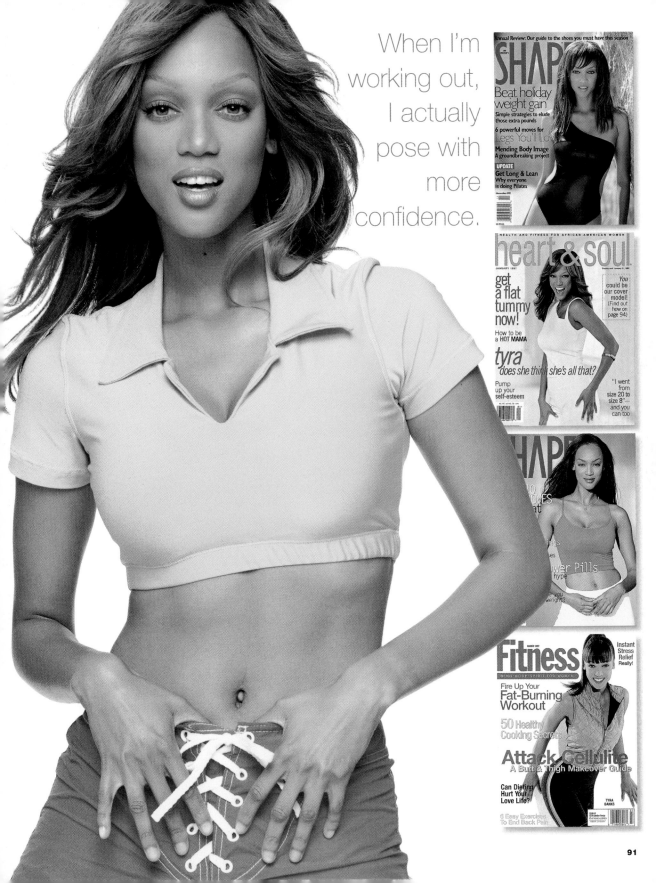

When I'm working out, I actually pose with more confidence.

ONE ON ONE

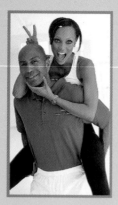

My trainer extraordinaire, Clayton James

I am always ready for a workout. I'm usually so eager that I bound out of bed in the morning, jump into my workout wear, and race to the gym so that I don't miss out on one minute of exercise time. NOT!!! The truth is, I get really lazy and lose focus. That's why I decided to get a personal trainer. With their high energy and expertise, personal trainers are an excellent source of motivation. They're also a good safeguard against injury, because they know the proper way the exercises should be done. They set a pace for you and make sure you aren't pushing yourself too hard or not enough.

I went through five or six personal trainers and a few frustrating months before I found just the right person: Clayton James. When I'm in New York, I work out with him five times a week, typically for one to two hours at a time. Because I get bored with doing the same thing day after day, we vary the routine. But whatever we do, Clayton makes sure that the four basic areas of fitness are covered: muscular strength, muscular endurance, flexibility, and cardiovascular work.

Before we start, I warm up my body with some light stretches. This is one step I won't blow off, because it helps me to loosen up my joints and improve my range of motion. Once I'm feeling limber, I do a three-mile jog on the treadmill. (Or, if the weather is nice, we'll run in the park.) After that, I stretch myself out again to make sure that I won't pull any muscles.

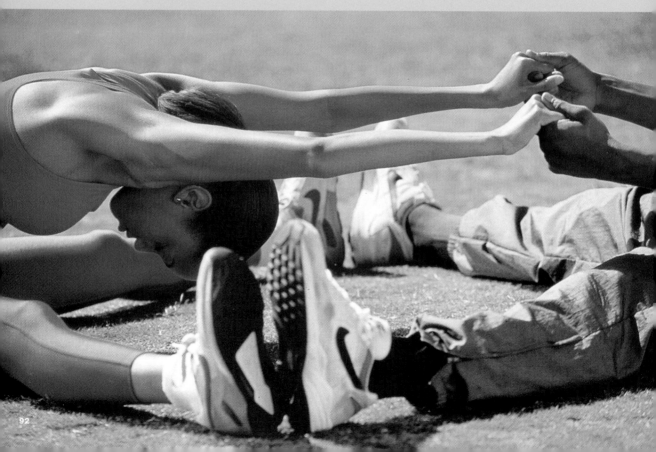

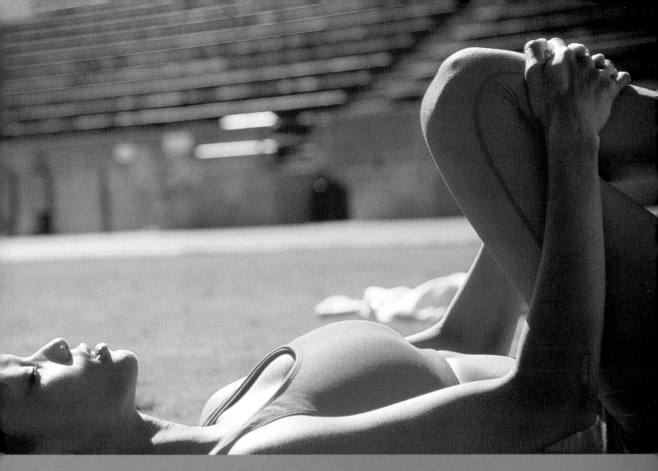

Then we move into strengthening the lower body. My target spots are my butt and upper thighs so we spend a lot of time working those areas. I do leg presses and leg extensions on the machines to work my gluteus maximus, thighs, and knees. Then we work the inner and outer thighs, and follow that with toe raises to work the calves. We also work on a machine we call the butt-master that attempts to keep my flabby backside firm.

We don't do everything on the machines, though. Clayton likes me to use my own body weight and ankle weights for resistance. We do squats and lunges, and then we'll do leg exercises such as donkey kicks with weights strapped on my ankles.

Next we focus on the mid body and work on my abdominals and back, using both ab machines and floor exercises such as sit-ups and crunches. Then we attack the lower back, which is where my stress seems to settle. I concentrate heavily on this area because I travel a lot, and sitting in cramped airplanes takes its toll.

The upper body is probably my weakest area. Clayton has me do push-ups, and chest-and-shoulder presses on the machine. But we also do a lot of work with free weights. Clayton says that the beauty of the free weights is that you can do more repetitions with a wider range of motion than you can with a machine.

With all the globe-trotting I do, it's hard to stay on a regular routine. I get lazy and start to skip my workouts. Clayton

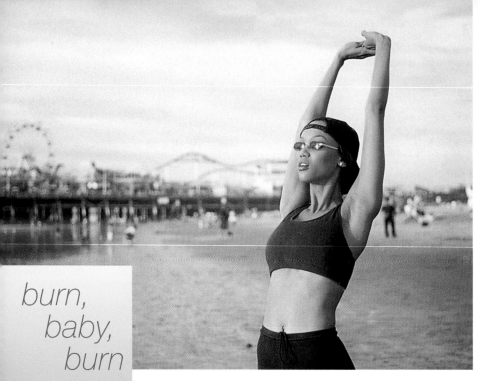

burn, baby, burn

Have you ever been exercising and felt a burning sensation in your legs that eventually goes away after an extended period of time? What you're experiencing may seem like torture, but it's actually lactic acid burn, a natural reaction that comes from doing repetitions, and it's good for you. You should exercise through the burn. If you stop as soon as you feel it, you won't get as good a workout.

However, if the burn feels like a pinch or pull, or doesn't go away, it may be a sign of injury. In this instance, you should stop exercising immediately and seek a doctor's advice. When in doubt, slow it down a bit until the burn stops.

calls me when I'm on the road or in L.A. to remind me to stick to my program and to give me a little push, which is a tremendous help. He also has me report back to him about the consistency of my workouts, and what I'm doing. Sometimes when I feel like I want to slack off, knowing that Clayton will be calling for a progress report is just the incentive I need to get going. His early-morning pep talks are a welcome wake-up call.

This kind of careful and concerned attention is exactly what makes for a good personal trainer. Trainers should be a walking, talking billboard for physical fitness. But they don't have to be all muscle-bound and look like Arnold Schwarzenegger either—just physically fit. They are there to do more than just crack the whip, though; they should also be willing to listen to your concerns. He or she should motivate you, be versatile, and vary the routine so that you don't get bored.

I know personal trainers aren't in everyone's budget, but there's a way of getting around the expense. The first time you visit a gym, invest in a one-time training session, and ask a trainer to walk you through all of the machines. As the trainer takes you through the equipment, record the information on a chart, so you can refer back to it whenever you need it. Once you get the hang of everything, you can do the workout on your own.

If having a personal trainer isn't an option, enlisting the help of a friend is a strong substitute. There are many days when I just don't feel like getting out of that warm, cozy bed to work out and get all sweaty. But then my buddy will call and say, "Tyra, get your tired butt up. I'm coming to pick you up right now and you'd better have on your workout clothes when I get there!"

I like the idea of having a group of workout partners because if one person drops out or loses interest, then you still have several others who can pick up the slack. The other good thing about working out with a group is that there is safety in numbers. It gives you another level of protection, especially when exercising outdoors.

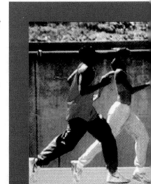

Get on Up

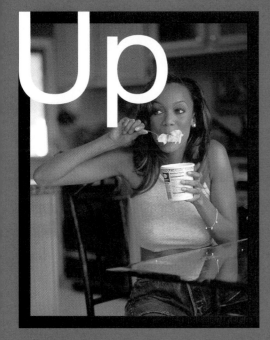

The other thing I like to do is exercise in front of my bedroom mirror with three- to five-pound hand weights, because I can actually see the muscle groups working.

If getting your butt out of the house to go to the gym is the problem, then make a nonrefundable appointment with your trainer, or a no-backing-out exercise date with a friend. Once I have that date set and circled in red in my day planner, I rarely break it. If the broken appointment is with my trainer, I can't get my money back. And if it's with my friend, she won't speak to me for a week.

I hear people say all the time that "I'd love to work out. I just don't have the time," but there's always time. Whether it's five minutes or thirty, that's enough to squeeze in some type of physical activity. Even on days when I can't complete an entire two-hour workout, I still try to fit something in. If I have only thirty minutes, I'll go into the gym and do some cardio-vascular work. If I have less time, I might go out and run an eight-minute mile. THERE'S ALWAYS TIME! You've just got to find it. And if you can't find the time, you've just got to make the time. Your body will thank you.

Your body will thank you.

A s I've said before, there are plenty of times when I'd rather be sitting up in bed eating some ice cream than in the gym with Clayton. But I try not to fall into that trap. Whenever I can, I introduce some pleasant touches into my routine, like listening to music with headphones, which makes working out more appealing. As I'm jogging along grooving to the music, occasionally I'll throw in a spontaneous dance step to shake things up. (But I never do this on a treadmill. Too dangerous.)

Go for the Goal

When you're getting fit, it helps to have a goal. It doesn't have to be anything elaborate—just attainable. Setting realistic goals is the first step toward success. Some other considerations:

Make sure that you enjoy the activity you've chosen. If you don't like to work out with other people, then an aerobics class is probably not the best option for you.

Set a time frame for what you hope to accomplish. Write it down and tell people if that helps you to stick with it. It makes your goals more concrete.

Don't be too hard on yourself. There are bound to be a few setbacks, such as low-energy days, a missed workout, or an injury. You may even have to rethink your game plan. The idea is not to dwell on that but to keep going.

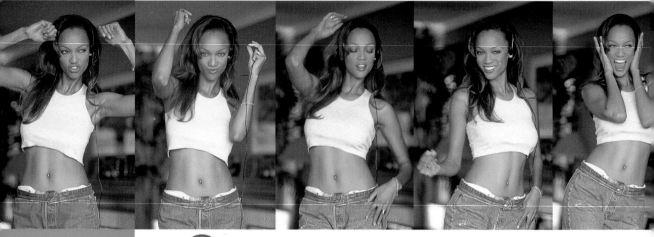

gr**OoV**E thang

I love running, but dancing is my all-time favorite workout. I grew up taking ballet and jazz-dancing lessons, which was lots of fun when I was a kid. But people don't realize that it can still be fun now. I once took an African dance class that made me work up a serious sweat, but hardly seemed like exercise at all. I walked in wearing a sports bra and sweatpants while everyone else wore colorful head and body wraps made of kente cloth to get into the mood, so of course I felt out of place. But when the live drummers began banging out the beat, I started to feel it deep down, and I danced and swayed to the rhythms. I had trouble keeping up with the class and was exhausted by the time it was over, but it sure did feel great afterward.

If you prefer a more private setting, crank up the CD player or tune the TV to your favorite music video station, close the bedroom door, and dance up a storm! While you're perfecting your moves, your arms, legs, buttocks, and abdominals will be getting a major workout.

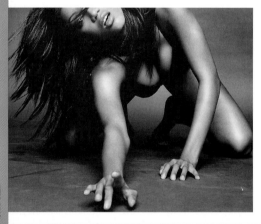

STAND UP STRAIGHT, GIRL!

When I was growing up, I was tall for my age and uncomfortable with my height. My parents, teachers, and even my bully of a brother were always telling me to "Stand up straight, girl!" Nowadays, if I do say so myself, my posture is A plus.

Playing it straight, instead of slouching, may seem a little stiff and formal to some. But in actuality, it's one of the best things you can do for your body. Good posture takes the pressure off the spine, pressure that can lead to lower back, leg, neck, and shoulder pain. It also creates the illusion of length, giving your body a nice, clean, vertical line. Standing tall is also a great image booster, because it projects self-confidence, no matter how you might feel on the inside. So stand up straight, girl.

You'll breathe easier, have more energy, exude confidence, and you'll look good too.

GAME TIME

On my mom's first day of school in the tenth grade, she tried out for the high school track team. Without having had any formal training, she went out for the long jump, and was such a natural talent that she unofficially broke her high school's records. The coach was so impressed, he was ready to sign her up right then and there! She was so excited that she ran all the way home to tell her mother the good news. But Grandma Florine nonchalantly took a puff from her cigarette and said, "That's very nice, baby, but your brother's already running track. Why don't you try something else, like dancing." The next day, Ma signed up for modern dance.

My grandmother's reaction was a sign of the times. Back then, there was a stigma attached to women in sports, and girls weren't encouraged to be strong and athletic. After my mom's experience, she promised herself that she would do things differently with her own daughter. So she encouraged me to try out for everything—basketball, volleyball, softball. And I was accepted on all the teams, because my coaches saw my five-feet, nine-inch height as an advantage—that is, until they saw me play.

I was so clumsy and uncoordinated that I eventually became the official bench-warmer.

When the coach finally did let me play in a volleyball match, I was so awkward that I sprained my forearm. When I made the basketball team, I couldn't shoot to save my life. So, unless we were way ahead or hopelessly behind, I didn't see much court time.

My dad refereed for the majority of the local Little League teams in our neighborhood and was a coach for my church's basketball squad, but that still didn't help me with my skills. I was a lost cause! But it didn't matter to him. He would still take me to Lakers games to influence me, thinking maybe some of Magic Johnson's power would rub off. It didn't work.

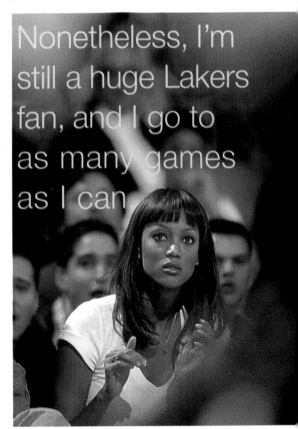

Nonetheless, I'm still a huge Lakers fan, and I go to as many games as I can.

Better yet, I get to watch the women tearing up the court now! It's great to see the divas of the WNBA, including Hai xia Xheng, Cynthia Cooper, and Teresa Weatherspoon, finally get their due. It's even more exciting to see young girls attending the games, sporting their Sparks, Comets, and Liberty jerseys, and getting all worked up and hyped as they watch the players. I get a lump in my throat every time I walk into the arena. These women are making history, breaking down barriers, and striking down stereotypes about women in sports. They are true pioneers and I'm proud to be there supporting them.

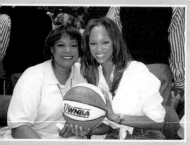

WNBA inaugural game, June 21, 1997

Today, women are playing almost every professional sport imaginable—even boxing! The power, grace, and energy of these athletes is inspirational. Anyone who's ever seen figure skater Michelle Kwan turn pirouettes in the air, watched Venus Williams take it to the net, or witnessed Amy Van Dyken slice through water at record speed knows what I'm talking about. With all this exposure, women are finally beginning to be taken a lot more seriously.

The presence of these new female pro athletes has had a major influence because more young girls and women are involved in sports than ever before. It's a move that makes sense. There is all kinds of evidence to prove that young women who participate in sports are healthier and more academically successful. They are less likely to drop out of high school and more likely to attend college. There are also a multitude of mind and body benefits. To name a few, sports participation increases cardiovascular endurance and strength, which decreases the chances of developing heart disease and high cholesterol. There is also evidence that sports promote self-esteem, mental toughness, and strong social skills.

With all this in our favor, there are still those who think it is inappropriate for a woman to break into a sweat. They have antiquated notions of what girls and women should—and should not—do, and playing sports is high on the list. I don't see how being athletic detracts from our femininity. A show of strength is just as feminine as a skirt and high heels.

How Ya Like Me Now?

Fortunately, with time and practice, my athletic skills have improved. Now I can dribble, block, and steal the basketball. But when it comes to shooting, it's time for me to pass it over to somebody else.

But whenever I'm feeling brave, I like to play basketball with the guys at the gym. Sometimes they try to ignore me, just to make me get frustrated and stop, but it never works. I remember one time I joined in on an all-guy pick-up game of volleyball, and I had to fight my way to getting recognized on the court. They did everything to prevent me from making contact with the ball. They would even run in front of me when the ball came right to me. So finally I just yelled, "You know, you need to stand back!" For the rest of the game, I didn't have any more problems. I even spiked on the other team a couple of times!

My biggest athletic challenge to date came a few years ago when I was in the movie *Higher Learning.* I played a woman who ran track for the college team. Track is about the only sport I didn't participate in in school, so I had absolutely no idea what to expect. Usually people have a couple of months to prepare for a movie. I had to learn how to hurdle in three weeks.

I worked out four hours a day, seven days a week, but thankfully I had a great trainer, Jeanette Bodin, the head women's track coach at UCLA. She's legit too, because she won a gold medal in the track relay in the 1984 Olympics.

When I first started training, my form was a little awkward, but I eventually got the hang of it. As soon as she felt I was ready, Jeanette decided that it was time for me to really start attacking the hurdles. I did fine the first couple of times. But on my third time around, I tripped over one of the hurdles and fell facedown on the ground. My hands and knees were bleeding from the gravel on the track, and my chest was so sore I thought I'd broken my ribs.

I was ready to call it a day, but Jeanette wouldn't let me. She had seen many runners go through the same thing, so she knew I wasn't hurt that badly. But I thought it was the end of the world. I was crying and rolling around on the track, dramatically gasping, "Oh, my ribs are broken, I can't do the movie, it's all over now." But she just said, "Get up, girl. Movie production hasn't started yet, so stop acting." She refused to let me quit. She said, "If you don't try again now, you'll never jump over the hurdles. You will have let them defeat you."

By then my ribs were feeling a little better, so I pulled myself up from the ground and started again. And my old crying-and-pleading self got over that hurdle. The approving smile on Jeanette's face made me hurdle five more. Up to when shooting started, I trained with her every day, and it was probably the hardest I've ever worked. Even though we wound up using a body double for those hurdling

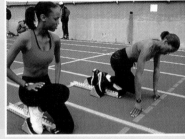

shots, it was a major achievement for me to have reached a place I couldn't have imagined being only three weeks before.

The only downside to the experience was that I'd started out full blast instead of slowly working my way up to that level. I was running so much that I lost twelve to fifteen pounds. Eventually I wound up getting a bad case of tendonitis in my ankles from all the intense training. It was a painful lesson—my ankles still crack from this. Now I know that no matter how physically fit you may feel, you should never rush. The risk of injury is too great.

The upside: When I thought I couldn't go on, I didn't quit. I think about that experience whenever something seems too difficult and I just want to give up. Ma always says never say "can't." Now I say, "I'll give it a try."

With women, physical fitness means more than just working out. We should also take care of those special needs that are uniquely feminine, such as our reproductive health.

Down Under

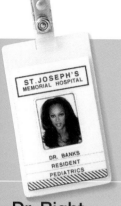

Dr. Right

Luckily, I have a gentle, caring physician who understands my concerns and reacts with care. Ideally, any doctor you choose should make you feel the same way. A good gynecologist will:

Explain everything in detail, and tell you step-by-step what is going to happen next.

Use sterilized tools and wear plastic gloves during the examination.

Answer all of your questions without intimidating you or making you feel foolish.

Involve you in the decision-making process by inviting a discussion.

Respect your confidentiality. Whatever's discussed in that exam room is between you and your doctor. But if it's super serious and life-threatening, others need to be notified.

For our reproductive well-being, all women should go for a yearly gynecological exam. I was about sixteen when my mother took me for my first checkup, and I was TERRIFIED. She told me exactly what the doctor was going to do before we went, so I knew what was going to happen, but I was just worried and nervous about having someone examine me "down there." I had never used tampons before (because I hadn't started to menstruate yet), and I wasn't sexually active, so I thought the examination would be painful. Since I was such a fraidy cat, my mom accompanied me into the examining room and held my hand during the visit.

Like many new experiences, it wasn't as bad as I'd expected. First, the doctor had me fill out some forms that asked about my medical history and some general questions about my health. Then she took my weight, and asked me to give her a urine specimen, to make sure everything was in balance.

My mom had warned me that I would have to remove all of my clothes and put on a thin paper robe, so I was mentally prepared for it. I just wasn't prepared for how cold it was in those rooms. Brrr! Then the doctor put on some plastic gloves, and the first thing she asked me to do was lie down on the examining table so that she could give me a breast exam. Since it was my first visit, she used a model of a woman's breast to show me how to do it, then she had me examine my breasts along with her so I would know what was normal and what wasn't. Thankfully, everything was fine.

Next, I had to put my legs in the air and my feet in stirrups so that she could do the pelvic exam. First, she lubricated a speculum and inserted it into my vagina so that she could get a good look inside. Then she did a Pap smear, which essentially means that she took a cotton swab and gently scraped the cervix for cell samples, which she sent to the lab to test for cancer and other diseases. When that was done, she removed the speculum. I have to say I did feel a little discomfort with that part, but with her and my mother chatting away, they both kept me so distracted that I barely noticed.

The last stage was a manual exam, where she inserted two fingers into my vagina to check my uterus and ovaries for any abnormalities. Then she inserted a finger into my rectum, also to check for unusual growths. Throughout the exam, she explained what she was doing so that I would understand the purpose for each step. I really appreciated that, because nothing took me by surprise.

The entire exam took no more than twenty minutes. Afterward, she told me to get dressed and we met her in her office, where she gave me a clean bill of health. By the next visit, I had started to menstruate, so we had more to talk about. But I felt so comfortable with her that I didn't have any problems discussing how long my menstruation lasted, or what the cramps were like. She's the one who helped me decide between tampons and pads. She explained that tampons were perfectly fine, as long as you didn't wear the same one for more than twelve- to fourteen-hour intervals. Because bacteria grows in a moist area, the body needs a break. She suggested switching over to pads at night.

As the years have gone on, we've also had discussions about my sexual history. It's all confidential, of course, so I don't worry. Like my gynecologist always says, "When you start to feel ashamed of yourself, that's when you're not going to get the best help for yourself."

Something Fishy's Going On

Vaginal infections are no fun, especially since they're usually accompanied by such a disturbing odor. But don't let it embarrass you. The smell is nature signaling to you that something is wrong.

Normally, every woman has her own natural vaginal smell. But certain circumstances can alter it. A yeast infection, for example, could be caused by a diet high in sugar, or a moist, enclosed environment, such as wearing pants that are too tight, or walking around all day in a wet bathing suit. It is usually accompanied by extreme itching and irritation, and a slightly medicinal smell. A bacterial infection, also known as bacterial vaginosis, could be caused by any bacteria that is introduced into your vagina. For example, bacteria may be carried in a man's semen and transmitted to you through sexual intercourse. Bacterial vaginosis has a foul, fishlike odor. (FYI, infections also change the color of your vaginal discharge from thin and whiteish or clear like egg whites, to yellow, green, or thick and white with a cottage-cheese consistency.)

How to get the odor in check? Whatever you do, don't try to mask it with a feminine deodorant spray, baby powder, or perfume. Douching is another no-no; the deodorants and/or chemicals might make matters worse. Instead, visit your doctor for an accurate diagnosis, especially if this is your first experience with an infection. She'll either prescribe a medication (if it's bacterial), or suggest an over-the-counter remedy (if it's yeast) to correct the problem. There are a range of seven-, three-, and one-day medications available in drugstores for yeast infections, and once you learn to recognize the symptoms, you can self-medicate.

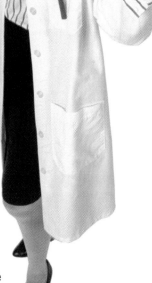

By the way, urinary tract infections are an entirely different issue. They're caused by bacteria that's pushed into the urethra or bladder areas, either through sexual intercourse or by wiping yourself from back to front instead of the reverse. Frequent and painful urination is one of the telltale signs that you have one. Treatment for urinary tract infections requires a doctor's visit. If not treated timely with antibiotics, the infection can move up into your kidneys, where it can be really serious.

Go with the Flow

Some women call it "the curse," others refer to it as "a visit from Aunt Flow," but whatever the code name, menstruation is a critical part of our reproductive health. It also influences the estrogen levels in the body. That's why it's so important to seek a doctor's help when we notice irregularities. It could simply be stress causing the problems, or it could be something a lot more serious.

Athletic types, in particular, should read the danger signs. Rigorous sports that result in low body fat, such as gymnastics and long-distance running, have been known to put a stop to menstruation. That may sound like heaven to some of you, but the temporary break can have harmful, long-term effects. These athletes are at greater risk for osteoporosis later in life, because their low fat-to-muscle ratio causes estrogen levels to drop, which then leads to a decrease in blood flow. This estrogen deficiency can lead to low bone density. So if you are experiencing anything abnormal, have a physician check it out.

Don't Sweat It

Throughout the book I've been talking about how great my mom is, how she's taught me so much, and how "together" she is. I have to admit that Ma is one helluva woman. She's been through it all (and I do mean all) and she's still going strong.

My mom is a superwoman. She'll pick up her toolbox (which rivals any man's) and personally perform all kinds of household repairs and maintenance on

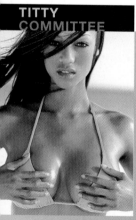

The media and the general public seem obsessed with my breasts: "Are they real or are they fake?" Whenever I go to the gynecologist for a breast exam, I tell her, "I wish you could televise this so the whole world could see I'm all natural." I used to joke and laugh and say the rumors didn't bother me, but they really do hurt my feelings. No matter what I say, people will believe what they want to believe, and I've just got to learn to live with that.

I'm more concerned with the health of my breasts than the hype. That's why I've gotten into the habit of examining my breasts on a monthly basis. I don't know why so many of us fail to do this. I guess there's a certain fear of the unknown, or perhaps we're afraid of finding something cancerous, or we could have the it-could-never-happen-to-me syndrome.

Before I started doing self-exams regularly, I used to be intimidated. I was afraid that I would not know what I was feeling for. I have large breasts that are fibrous (clusters of thick tissue that can feel like lumps), so it makes it harder to detect any differences, and that worried me.

But then I talked to my doctor about it, and she told me that the more I got to know my breasts by examining them on a regular basis, the better I would be able to distinguish between normal fibrous tissue and any irregularities. So now I follow the guidelines health professionals recommend and look for lumps once a month.

The best time to do it is about a week after your period has begun, when hormonal changes are the least likely to affect your breasts. Some people examine themselves in the shower, but I prefer to lie down with one hand behind my head, leaving the other hand free to do the exam. I mimic the way my doctor examines my breasts: she presses down with the pads of her fingers in a clockwise direction. It really doesn't matter which direction you start in, just as long as you follow the same pattern throughout the exam so you don't miss anything. What you're looking for are any unusual masses, swelling, puckering, redness, or soreness. I do this on both breasts, and then I check the tissue underneath the armpits for the least likely to affect anything out of the ordinary.

My last step is to stand in front of the mirror with my arms raised above my head to see if the shape of my breasts has changed in any way. I also squeeze my nipples to check for any discharge.

The entire thing takes only about five minutes. That five minutes could save your life.

Three things we think are weird about our breasts but are actually perfectly normal:

1. one is larger than the other
2. inverted nipples
3. hairs around the aureole

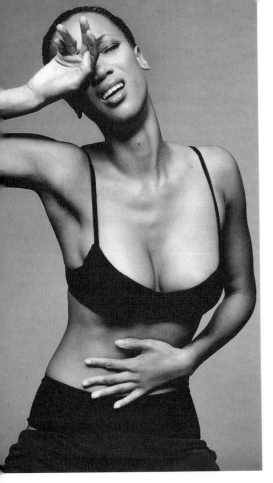

around the time of day when the "peppy rabbit" turns into a "snapping turtle."

What my mother–and many of us–sometimes forget is how much our mental health affects our physical health. If we aren't careful to control them, the stresses in our lives can cause fatigue, backaches, headaches, and other physical ailments.

While we may all joke sometimes about Ma's hyperenergy, deep down inside, her behavior makes me extremely nervous and worried about her health. I've taken several measures to relieve her from a lot of the pressure by making her disconnect her pager, put away the cellular phone, and close up the laptop; then I've shipped her off somewhere, forcing her to take minivacations through-out the year. I've also been trying to teach her how to say "NO!" I haven't been too successful. Wish me luck.

Stress is a part of life. We have to accept the fact that it's not going to go away. The trick is to learn how to deal with it in a healthy way.

We are living in a momentous age, where the roles of women in all areas are growing and expanding. That's why it's important that we take time to pay attention not only to how our bodies look, but how we feel about them. When we are able to attain a state of well-being with ourselves, both physically and mentally, we are well-equipped to meet all of life's challenges head-on and healthily.

Four Ways to Squash Stress

1. Face your problems head-on: I always mistakenly tell my mom to *just forget* about her problems and hectic schedules. But it's important to look every-thing squarely in the face so you can deal with it directly.

2. Work it out: Exercising is an excellent stress reducer. Trying to hike up a super-steep hill or run an eight-minute mile will make your problems seem a lot easier in comparison.

3. Relax your mind: Meditating will give you an opportunity to really be alone with your thoughts. It also has health benefits, because it relaxes your muscles and slows down your heart rate.

4. Insist on a list: Formulate, systemize, coordinate–writing down what you need to do, especially when stressed, is a sure way to calm your nerves. It clears your mind of all those jum-bled thoughts running through your head.

my house and hers! She loves gardening, has singlehandedly hauled ten-gallon tubs of plants up the hillside of her home, and she has dutifully managed my career for the past six years.

Need a helping hand? Advice or coun-seling? Having a family crisis? Want to build a skyscraper? Why not just call Carolyn? Her hands are always full, but she'll somehow make room for just one more project. She may almost kill herself in the process, but she always gets the J-O-B done. She just doesn't know when to say "NO," so she is constantly pushed to the max. When she is stressed, she doesn't just get a little tired and take a short rest. She just keeps on running like the Energizer bunny until her batteries run out. This is usually

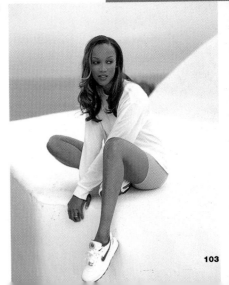

103

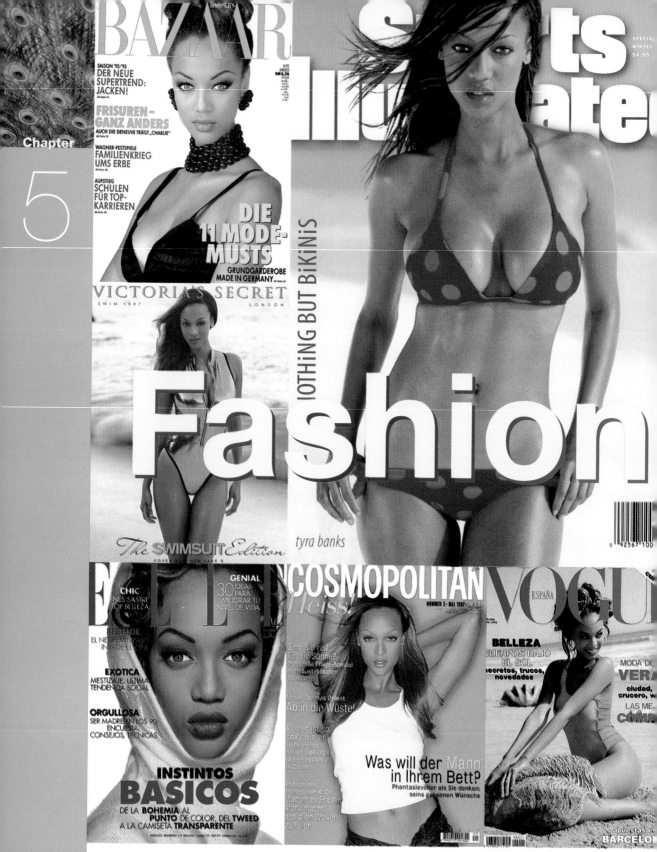

Summer Springs.

That's what my buddies Sam and Oscar call me because I always wear warm-weather clothes, no matter what the season or weather forecast. It could be snowing in New York, and I'd still have on a halter top, short shorts, and some flip-flops – I'd just throw a big winter coat over it. Blame it on my hometown. The sun is always shining in sunny Los Angeles, California, so I'm used to dressing in clothing designed for a warm climate. And I'm not about to change that just because I've crossed a few state lines!

I guess I've always been sort of a nonconformist when it comes to fashion. I sported the grunge look long before it was trendy. When I first started modeling in Paris, I wore an oversize T-shirt with baggy overalls, combat boots, and a fishing cap. And I carried my high school backpack with my portfolio of pictures to all of my interviews at various magazine headquarters and designer showrooms (in the modeling industry, it's okay to wear street clothes to an interview). Most of the other models were wearing black, fitted dressy tops, black leggings, and black ankle boots with three-inch heels, and they all carried black name-brand satchels to hold their portfolios. That seemed to be the standard uniform. But I couldn't understand how they could run around the city from appointment to appointment all day long, usually on the subway, in confining clothes and heels.

Instead of trying to look like the rest of them, I just did my own thing.

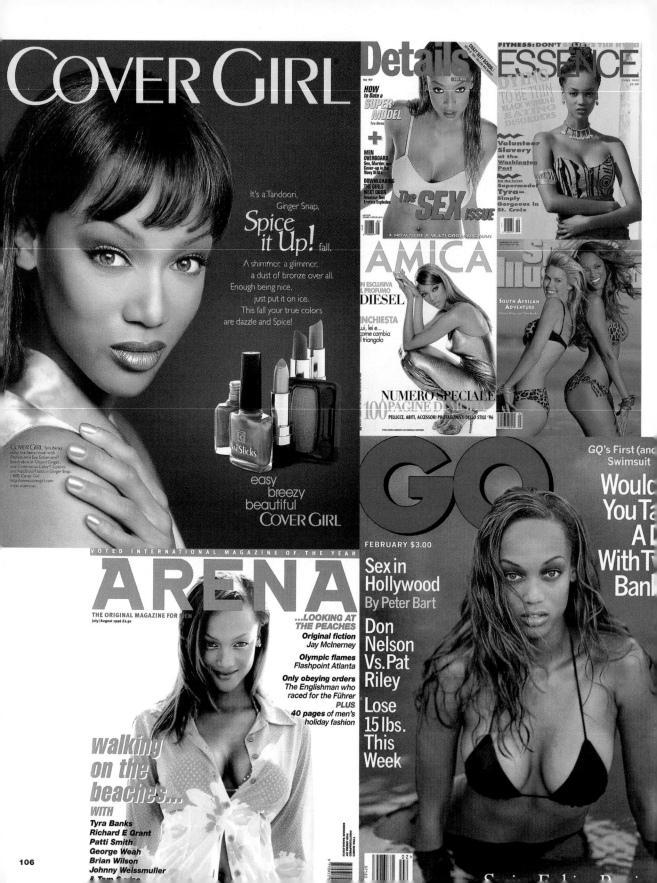

Details

May 1997

HOW
to Date a
**SUPER
MODEL**
Tyra Banks

+

MEN
OVERBOARD
Sex, Murder, and
Cover-up in the
Navy SEALs

DOWNLOADING
THE GIRLS
NEXT DOOR
Amateur Net
Erotica Explodes

The **SEX** issue

+ HOW TO BE A MULTI-ORGASMIC MAN

FITNESS: DON'T BELIEVE THE HYPE

ESSENCE

JUNE 1993

TO BE THIN
BLACK WOMEN &
EATING
DISORDERS

Volunteer
Slavery
at the
Washington
Post

On the Cover:
Supermodel
Tyra—
Simply
Gorgeous in
St. Croix

AMICA

IN ESCLUSIVA
IL PROFUMO
DIESEL

INCHIESTA
Lui, lei e...
come cambia
il triangolo

NUMERO SPECIALE

100 **PAGINE DI MODA**

PELLICCE, ABITI, ACCESSORI PROTAGONISTI DELLO STILE '96

SOUTH AFRICAN
ADVENTURE

Valeria Mazza and Tyra Banks

VOTED INTERNATIONAL MAGAZINE OF THE YEAR

ARENA

THE ORIGINAL MAGAZINE FOR MEN
July/August 1996 £2.50

...LOOKING AT
THE PEACHES

Original fiction
Jay McInerney

Olympic flames
Flashpoint Atlanta

Only obeying orders
The Englishman who
raced for the Führer
PLUS
40 pages of men's
holiday fashion

**walking
on the
beaches...**
WITH

**Tyra Banks
Richard E Grant
Patti Smith
George Weah
Brian Wilson
Johnny Weissmuller**

GQ

GQ's First (and
Swimsuit

FEBRUARY $3.00

**Sex in
Hollywood**
By Peter Bart

**Don
Nelson
Vs. Pat
Riley**

**Lose
15 lbs.
This
Week**

Would
You Ta
A D
With T
Ban

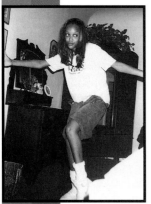

I guess my bummy fashion approach set me apart from the crowd and made a big impression on the designers. That first season in Paris, I was booked for a record-breaking twenty-five fashion shows in a six-day period, which up to that point was unheard of for a newcomer.

It just goes to show you that fashion is what you make it. Anybody can buy the latest and newest. It's the personal stamp you put on an outfit that really sets you apart. So, I follow fashion, but I'm not a slave to it.

All my years spent in private school had a major influence on my attitude toward clothes. We had to wear uniforms every day, so I rarely got the chance to put together outfits on my own. In elementary school, we wore blue jumpers with red-and-blue-striped belts. In high school, we were given a little more leeway to do some improvising. We could choose between two skirts, either gray wool in winter or yellow cotton in the spring, alternate between three shirt colors (blue, yellow, or white), and wear either penny loafers or oxfords.

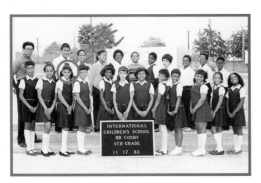

During those years, I got used to the school board dictating what I had to wear. Their influence even spilled over into my weekend wear: I created another kind of uniform—plain old jeans and a white T-shirt.

After I graduated from high school and started globe-trotting for various modeling jobs, I was exposed to different ways of dressing. I studied how women in other countries did it. I was most taken with the women of Africa and their way of using classic kente cloth fabrics. Some wore them as beautiful head wraps, while others draped them stylishly over the shoulder to accentuate a business suit.

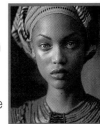

I was bombarded with so many incredible ideas that I began to think of dressing as a means of creative expression, not a dull routine. I began to loosen up some of my own rules and let go of the restrictions that had held me back from trying new things. Once I had the opportunity to wear whatever I wanted, I was like a kid in a candy store, sampling here, experimenting there. Now my closet is full of a little bit of everything—vintage, sexy and slinky, tailored and classic looks.

I will admit though that despite this great wardrobe I've built up, my old standbys frequently call to me, and more often than not, I've got jeans on my body. Only now, I vary the T-shirt colors: pink, mint green, brown, or baby blue.

I guess some things never change.

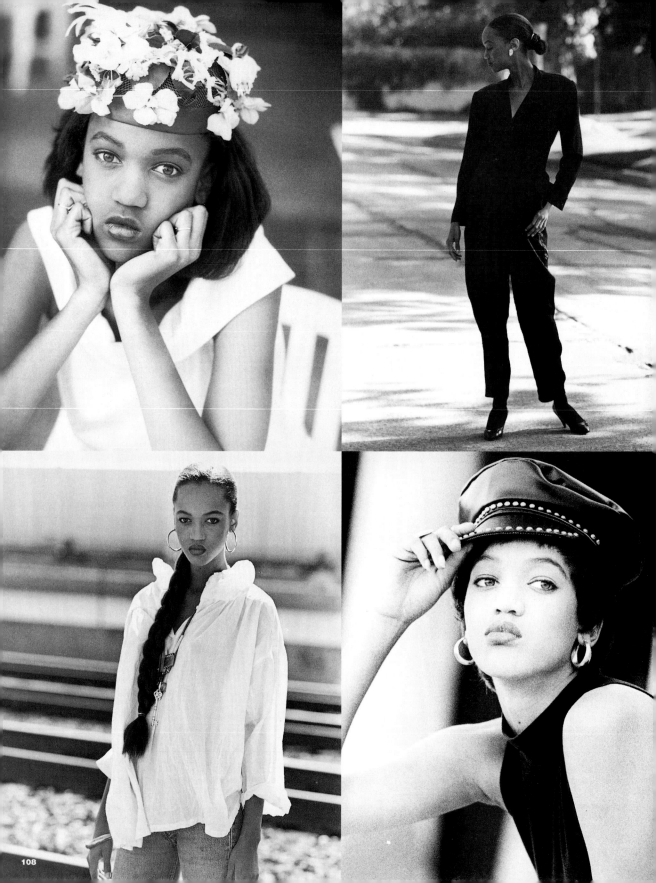

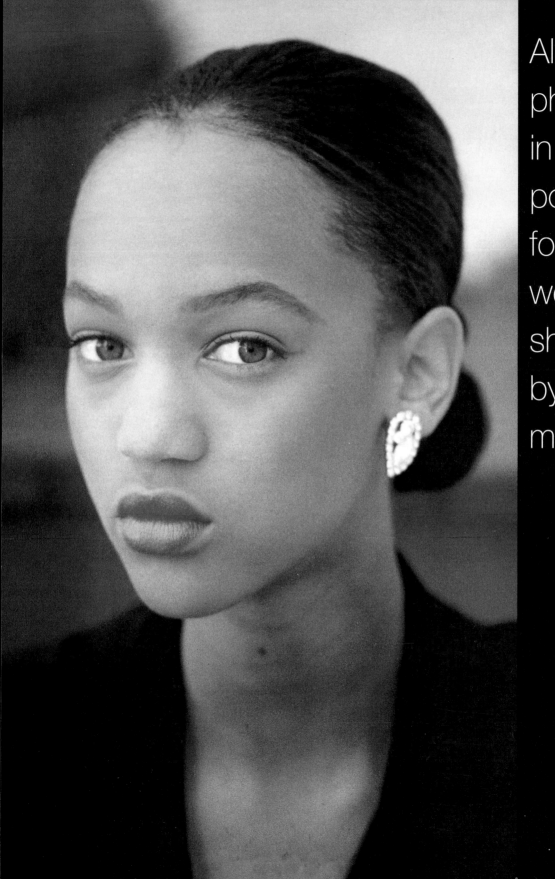

All the photos in my portfolio for Paris were shot by my mom.

Under the Influence

People say that models are trendsetters, that their personal style usually sets the pace, and that the public follows them. That's true to a certain extent, because when you are surrounded by clothes day after day, it's easy to know your way around a clothing rack. I've always envied models who can put together that perfect outfit.

Too bad that savvy never rubbed off on me. If imitation is the most sincere form of flattery, then I've lavished praise on all kinds of women over the years—the girl at a nightclub with the slinky slip dress; the businesswoman who turned heads in her man-tailored suit; the down-to-earth actress famous for her simple, pared-down elegance. I register these looks in my mental Rolodex and whenever I feel that my look needs a jolt, I pull them out for inspiration.

And yes, I look at magazines too for ideas on how to pull an outfit together. There are some magazines that outline step-by-step what pieces to buy, right down to the accessories. I clip and save

the pages I like and sometimes bring them with me to the mall as a quick reference guide. I need all the help I can get.

As I said before, Oscar and Sam are constantly ragging on me because I am such a fashion misfit. But I do have my moments. I can pull together an evening outfit just like a professional stylist, from handbag to heels. For most other occasions, however, I rely on a team of hairdressers, makeup artists, and fashion stylists to help put me together. They're great sources of advice because they are on the pulse of what's happening.

The same goes for any of your stylish friends: Ask them where they shop or go along on their next shopping spree. They're sure to be flattered—as long as you don't buy the exact same outfit. Not many people want to walk around looking like a twin (unless, of course, you are one).

The one place where I do feel totally at home: interior design. People who come to my house are always surprised that I'm the one who did all the decorating. Now, if I could only carry over that design sense into my wardrobe…

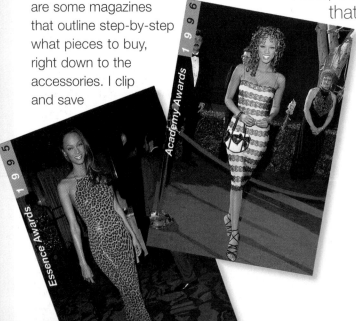

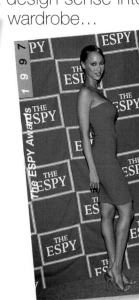

110

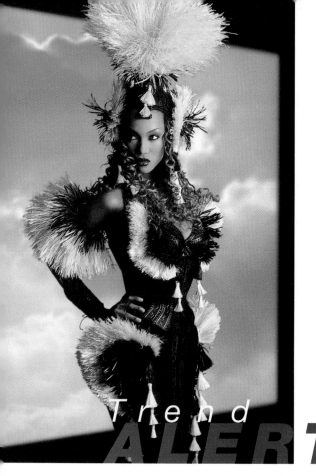

Trend
ALERT

But Ma knew that the outfit would probably be collecting dust in the back of my closet before the season was over. So instead of the designer brand, she would buy me a look-alike that was just as cool, but less expensive than the original. I'd go to school on free-dress day, showing off my knockoffs, and no one knew the difference.

Fashion is so fickle. The trendiest and hottest looks go in and out of style so quickly, it's hardly worth spending large sums of money on items that won't survive beyond this fleeting fashion moment. If it's important to you to be on the cutting edge, invest in the latest in **a small way.**

The 1980s: big hair, heavy makeup, and wild, flashy, and colorful clothes. During the height of this era, I was ten years old and highly impressionable. Once a month at school, we had "free-dress day" when we didn't have to wear a uniform, and there was always a big competition among the girls to see who had on the latest threads. So if there was a look that everyone else had except poor little ol' me, I would beg my mother to buy it for me. I just *had* to have that fluorescent green shorts set, Madonna lace crop top with matching gloves, and Jennifer Beals's *Flashdance* gear. I would literally get on my hands and knees and hound and hound her until she finally said yes.

COLOR Struck

When I first started buying clothes for myself, I got stuck in a color rut. Every time I went shopping, I'd come back with only basic, neutral shades. If I was feeling really adventurous, I would throw in a little navy blue. Before I knew it, I had a closet full of brown, black, and gray pieces. It was very reminiscent of my school uniform days.

It's good to have neutrals in your wardrobe as a foundation. But like they say, variety is the spice of life. Those subdued shades of mine got old pretty quickly, especially after I saw how great bright colors looked on my buddy Kenya. She is practically addicted to vibrant orange, candy-apple red, taxicab yellow, and kiwi green, and says neutrals do absolutely nothing for her. Now when I think of it, she was kind of in a rut herself, just the opposite of mine. But then one day I talked her into wearing a chocolate-brown dress, and she looked absolutely gorgeous! So the lesson here is clear: **Don't knock it if you haven't tried it.**

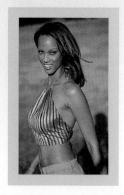

Dress for Success

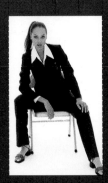

When I was looking for a personal assistant last year, I interviewed a bunch of candidates, and I couldn't believe the way some people dressed for their appointments. Some people came in as if they'd just spent a day at the beach; others dressed in very casual, almost hippielike clothes.

You know they say you can't judge a book by its cover, yet I couldn't help but think that if this is the way these people would show up for a job interview—casual, overly relaxed—then I could probably expect the same of their work habits. Now there's nothing wrong with being an individual and wanting to stand out from the crowd. But unless you know for certain that a little creativity is acceptable (like the freedom I had when I went on those Paris interviews), it's best to leave the quirkiness at home.

When you're in the job market, what you wear to the interview is your calling card. Many employers make up their minds about you in the first few minutes, so you want to make those moments count.

Just when I was about to throw in the towel for the day, in walked Debra Jackson.

She wore a simple suit with a classic silk scarf tied around her neck, and she looked like she meant business. Debra had left nothing to chance. Her makeup was subtle and understated and flattering to her face. And her neck scarf was a nice way of adding a personal touch. She respected the fact that this was a professional encounter and that she was expected to dress appropriately. Of course, she had the credentials to back up the look too. So, I guess it's pretty obvious— she got the job!

What's funny is that her true style is relaxed and easy. But she saved that until *after* she was hired. Smart woman.

Adventures
in the Fitting Room

A few years ago, I was shopping at a mall in Los Angeles and went into the fitting room of a trendy store to try something on. I had stripped down to just my panties, when all of a sudden the saleswoman swung open the door to my stall and screamed,

"Wow, it really is Tyra Banks!"

Needless to say, the entire store heard her, and before I could grab for my clothes, I had about twenty-four inquiring eyes staring at me. And I could just imagine what they were thinking: "Oh, yes, that is *definitely* Tyra Banks—in the flesh!" I felt exposed to the world. But thank God no one had a camera. I'd probably be in court right now trying to stop the photos from being published.

As embarrassing as that experience was for me, it hasn't stopped me from trying things on in a store before I take them home. In the past, I've blown too much money trusting my eyes to sell me on an item, only to get it home and find out that the armholes are too deep and I can see my bra, or a jacket's shoulders make me look like a linebacker, or the pants legs are so short that I look like I've already outgrown them—and they're brand new! I've definitely learned my lesson.

Ma, however, is still working on it. She is the return and exchange queen! She hates to try on anything in the store, so she's always got some merchandise sitting in the trunk of her car—still in the shopping bag—that has to go back to the store because it doesn't fit. I've started calling her the "bag lady."

No matter how much of a rush I'm in, and just want to grab something and go, I force myself to take a few minutes to visit the fitting room. Based on my experiences, I've come up with some pointers that'll hopefully make the try-on process as painless as possible for you:

Before I leave the house on a shopping trip, I make sure I'm dressed in clothes that are easy to change out of, such as sundresses or stretch pieces that won't easily wrinkle. I also make sure there aren't a "bazillion" buttons to deal with.

When I'm in a department store, I'll wait in line a bit longer if I can get the fanciest fitting room in the store. They're usually well lit and twice as large as those dull, drab, shoebox-size rooms. And most have three-way mirrors that allow me to see what I look like from the back and all sides. (But I hope they don't have any surveillance cameras behind those mirrors. I spend so much time in there posing and goofing and having fun that I almost forget what I went in there to do.) Typically, there's also a chair inside the stall so you can check how well a skirt or pair of pants fits when you sit.

Cosmetics can make a mess of whatever you're trying on, so I usually skip wearing any makeup.

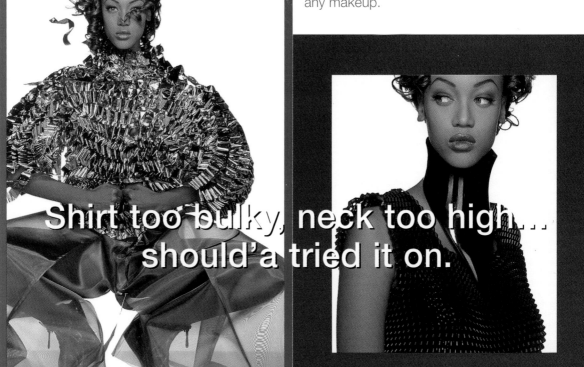

Shirt too bulky, neck too high... should'a tried it on.

GO FIGURE

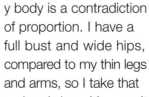

My body is a contradiction of proportion. I have a full bust and wide hips, compared to my thin legs and arms, so I take that into consideration when I shop. You won't catch me in a pair of white stretch pants because I have some cellulite, which I know isn't necessarily a horrible thing. It's natural and a lot of women have it. But unless I'm wearing a bathing suit, I'd rather keep it to myself. I usually wear dark-colored pants with a boot-cut or straight leg—anything tapered, like leggings, draws too much attention to my skinny calves. To accommodate my full bust, I prefer to wear tops with darts, otherwise I look top-heavy. And forget about fishtail-style dresses—they make my hips look out of proportion to the rest of my body, sort of like the distortion mirror in a funhouse, so I stay away from them.

Since I like my waistline, I often accentuate it with crop tops. I'm pretty partial to my collarbone too, so it's rare that you'll catch me wearing a turtleneck. V necks, boat necks, or any style that showcases the neckline works for me.

Some women have shapely legs, some have a flattering bustline, others have satiny shoulders and a smooth back; everyone has an asset worth highlighting. What do you love about you? Is it your long, graceful neck, defined arms, curvy hips, toned calves, or round behind?

Find it, and flaunt it!

Quality IQ

As a teen, I used to buy everything dirt cheap. That was my claim to fame! I'd get my clothing allowance, and stretch it to the max, then brag to my friends about the ten shirts I bought for $100. But then I'd get the shirts home, wear them once, and they'd fall apart after one washing. I'd have to wave good-bye to $100 as it went down the washing machine drain.

After that happened a few times, I began to get wiser about how I spent my money. Learning to recognize quality is the first step in shopping smart, especially when you're making a major investment. But remember that a higher price doesn't necessarily mean higher quality. Before you step up to the cash register, give the garment a good once-over. Here's what to look for:

Check the seams for loose threads, openings, or uneven stitching.

Look for a lining. Well-made jackets, pants, and skirts will have one. Linings make fabrics fall nicely and prevent wrinkles, and also help keep the shape of the garment.

If the shirt has darts, they should not fall above the bustline.

Do the tug test. Check for loose or missing buttons so you won't have to race for the sewing kit when you get home.

Feel the material. Grab a handful and rub it gently. If the material lacks substance, or is sheer but is not meant to be see-through, then it's probably best to pass it up.

Make sure zippers can move up and down easily without being forced.

If a garment passes all of these tests, it's safe to say you'll be making a good buy.

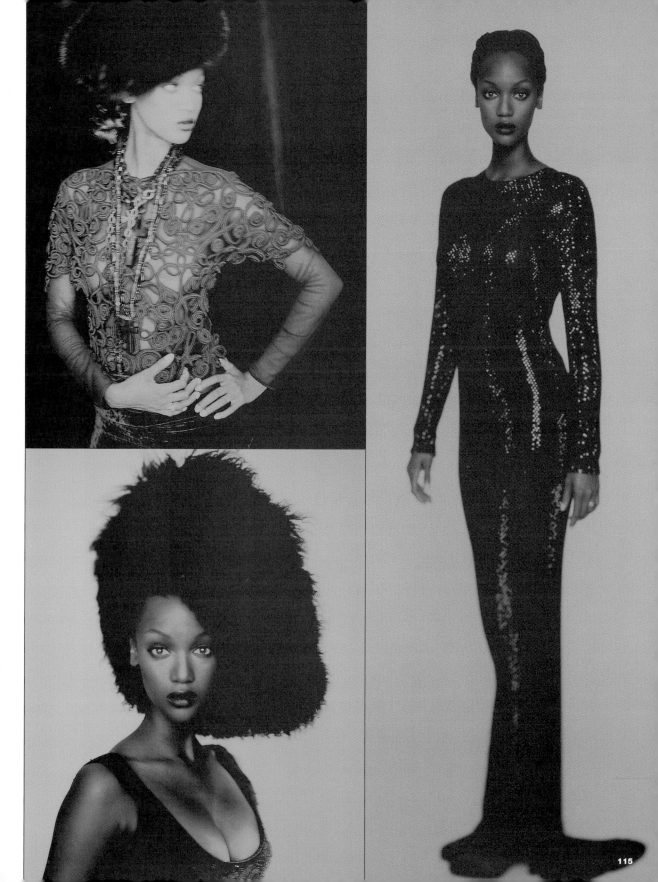

Tailor-Made

Going to an all-girls high school made any event involving the male species cause for all kinds of commotion. So of course the senior prom was a huge deal—the girls would start planning their outfits months in advance! I spotted the dress I wanted in an Italian magazine. It was a classic Jackie O style, designed by one of the top three Italian designers in the world, so you know it cost a pretty penny. I showed my mom the picture and told her that that was the dress I wanted. She took one look at the price and shouted, "Hey, time out Miss Moneybags!"

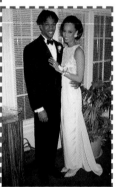

Instead, we took the idea to a seamstress and had the dress made. We bought a fabric similar to the one in the picture, and no one at that prom could tell the difference. They all thought I had spent a fortune!

Some people have a knack for home sewing. They just pick out a pattern, buy some material, and they've got an original design at the touch of a needle. I was not blessed with such skills, so I hand over the stitching to a seamstress or a tailor.

Recently I tried to save a favorite sundress that I had worn so much it was falling apart. So I took it to a master seamstress, Linda Stokes, to see if it could be altered. The dress was beyond repair, so instead, she drew up a pattern and made an *exact* copy of the dress. Then she used that same pattern to make a skirt and top for me in another color. Now, instead of getting rid of an item because it doesn't fit perfectly, I'll ask her to do a little nip and tuck on it. And, like the seamstress who made my prom dress, Linda is so skilled that she can make an outfit from a photograph and have it look just like the original.

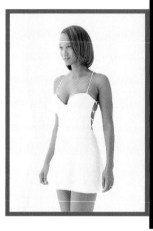
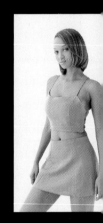

Tailors and seamstresses are especially good when you want a designer look at an affordable price. As for basics such as an A-line skirt, you'd probably be better off buying right off the rack. The following are a few more things to consider before you decide to have an item custom-made:

Tailors specialize in suits. Seamstresses deal primarily with dresses and more intricate designs. Both are good at alterations. If you're having something made, using quality fabric will result in a longer-lasting garment.

Get a good recommendation from someone you trust or ask to see samples of someone's work. Not everyone who hangs out a storefront sign is reputable.

Booby Trap

Before I started modeling, I never really paid much attention to my lingerie. One bra was as good as another. Or so I thought. After spending so much time around every bra imaginable in my work as a contracted spokesmodel for Victoria's Secret, I think I've become a semipro in the brassiere business.

You wouldn't believe how many times people have consulted me for a little lingerie advice, and sometimes even approval! Once when I was traveling, a flight attendant was so eager to show me that she had ordered one of the bras I modeled in the catalog that she opened her shirt and gave me a peep show right there on the plane in front of everybody! What could I do? I told her it looked nice and she went back to helping the other passengers as if nothing had happened. (Actually, the fit was pretty good.)

Finding a bra that measures up is really a matter of trial and error. There are so many varieties on the market, and there's so little consistency in sizing. A 34C in one brand could be a 36C in another. As we get older, our breasts change, so the bra that fit us when we were eighteen may be entirely wrong for us at thirty. According to some experts, at least 70 percent of women are wearing the wrong bra size. I have a friend who used to wear a 34B until she was properly measured and found out that she was actually a 36C. Her body had the strap marks and bruises to prove it.

Victoria's Secret and a number of department stores have people on staff who know how to measure breast size. Actually, it's a quick and easy process. A saleswoman will take you into a fitting room and, using a tape measure, figure out your back width and bust size in inches. From these measurements, she can gauge your cup size and what type of bra will give you a comfortable fit. And, best of all, it's doesn't cost anything.

These women are such professionals that you shouldn't feel the least bit uncomfortable having one see you topless. But if you're too shy to bare all in front of a stranger, here are a couple of ways in the privacy of your own home to make sure that your bra fits perfectly:

Beware of boob bulge. A bra should not cut into the top of your breasts. If it does, you'll look like you have four breasts instead of two.

Give your back a break. If you have a wide back, an extender can be attached to your back strap to stretch it out and ease the tension.

Avoid the tight squeeze. If a bra strap is cutting into your shoulders or the underwire is digging into your ribs, the bra is most likely either too small or is not cut to fit your contours.

a Shoe-in

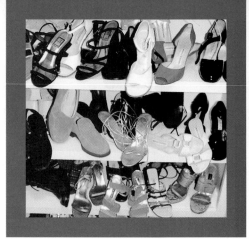

I f you were to take a peek inside my closet, you would see instantly what my weakness is: SHOES. I don't know what it is—I can't seem to walk through the shoe department without stopping. And don't let there be a sale—I'm in heaven! I guess buying different styles of shoes is more fun than wearing them, though, because I'm usually seen in sneakers or flip-flops. Whenever I announce that I'm clearing out my shoe collection, every size-9 ½ woman within a thirty-mile radius comes over to collect.

But even if I don't wear every single pair of shoes I own, you can bet they are all comfortable. I read somewhere that nine out of ten women still wear shoes that are too small for their feet. There is no reason a woman should have to suffer for fashion's sake. It's difficult for me to find shoes because I have a long and extremely narrow foot, size 9 ½ with a AAA width. Many stores now offer attractive styles in large, narrow, and wide sizes, and there are even specialty stores where you can have shoes custom-made. Of course, the style and expense of the shoes you sport is all a matter of taste, but fit is one area in which you shouldn't settle. A few footnotes on finding a good fit:

Have your feet measured regularly; they grow with age.

Shop at the end of the day, when feet are largest.

Bring your own hosiery. You don't know who's been walking around in those Peds the shoe department always has lying around.

Thick socks are another no-no when trying on a dressy pump or other shoe that isn't compatible with them. Try to wear socks or hosiery that suit the style you're shopping for.

Make sure the widest part of your foot measures up with the widest part of your shoe. This eliminates bunions and corns.

Don't stop after trying on only one of the shoes in the box. Just because one fits fine doesn't mean they both do. To be sure, it's best to take them both for a test drive.

Surf's Up

Ever since I posed for the *Sports Illustrated* swimsuit covers, people think I'm a swimwear expert. I've certainly picked up a wealth of knowledge about what's out there, especially the range of special features—bust enhancers, waist nippers, hidden control panels—and styles such as thong- and Brazil-cut bottoms, even suits whose makers claim their designs allow you to tan right through the suit without leaving tan lines.

But a pro I'm not. I just know what I like. My favorite look is the triangle-cut bikini,

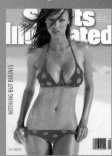

like the style I wore on last year's cover of *SI*. But I think one-piece styles can also look great. The key to finding the right suit is knowing your body and the features you want to play up. Whatever your figure, there's a style out there to flatter you.

Buggin' Out

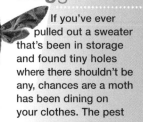

If you've ever pulled out a sweater that's been in storage and found tiny holes where there shouldn't be any, chances are a moth has been dining on your clothes. The pest problem is easy to correct. Just place some mothballs, cedar blocks, or cedar chips in your storage area. The chemicals they contain should ward off the "enemy" and keep your clothes totally intact. (To avoid other unsightly surprises such as stains and body odor, it's generally a good idea to have clothes cleaned before you store them for the season.)

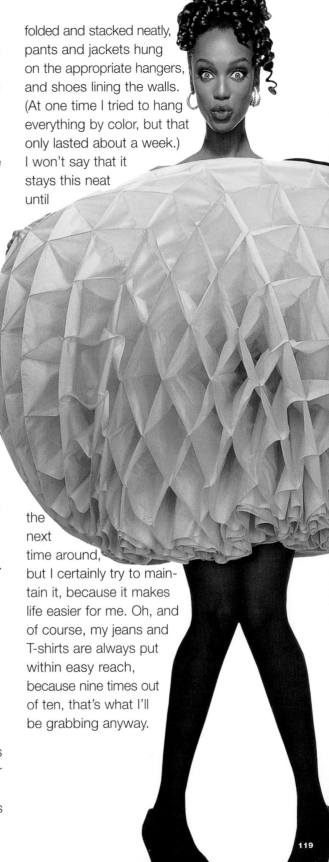

Whenever my closet gets so crowded that I can't find what I need when I need it, that's my cue to start reorganizing. I wait so long that it usually takes me all day to whip it back into shape, but it's well worth the time and effort because the cleanup keeps my wardrobe fluid and functional.

A friend once told me that if you haven't worn something for an entire year, it doesn't belong to you anymore; give it to someone who will wear and appreciate it. So, the first thing I do is dig all the way into the recesses of my closet to see what's hiding back there. Usually, it's either clothes that need some kind of alterations or impulse purchases that still have the price tags on them. As I pull them out, I create four piles: one of clothes that need to be tailored, a second one of clothes that need some kind of coordinates (a matching skirt, jacket, pants, etc.), a pile of never-to-be-worn-agains that I give to my little cousins or donate to charity, and, last, a pile of keepers. All of this includes my shoes and accessories as well.

The cardinal rule of cleaning out your closet is that you have to BE HONEST with yourself. Even if that skirt you've been holding on to for five years does come back in style, are you *really* going to wear it? If you have to stop and think about it, the answer is probably no.

The last–but most crucial–step in my closet check is putting each piece in its proper place. I group everything together by category–summer dresses in one section, workout clothes in another, shirts folded and stacked neatly, pants and jackets hung on the appropriate hangers, and shoes lining the walls. (At one time I tried to hang everything by color, but that only lasted about a week.) I won't say that it stays this neat until the next time around, but I certainly try to maintain it, because it makes life easier for me. Oh, and of course, my jeans and T-shirts are always put within easy reach, because nine times out of ten, that's what I'll be grabbing anyway.

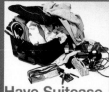

Have Suitcase, Will Travel

A few tricks I've picked up on the road:

Wrap any clothes that are easily wrinkled in tissue paper or plastic (those dry-cleaner bags are perfect) before you pack them up. It keeps creases from forming. Condense toiletries into small containers, then place them in sealable plastic bags. The pressure in airplane cabins tends to make bottles expand and spill out all over the suitcase. Put shoes in shoe bags or plastic bags before you pack them away, or you run the risk of getting dirt from the soles of your shoes all over your clothes. (Shoes also make great storage space for items such as a small camera because they protect whatever's sitting inside.) Don't overpack. Bring along just enough for your needs, and if you run out of clean clothes while you're away, do a small load of laundry. Bring your breakables with you in your carry-on luggage. If you check them in with the rest of your luggage, they could crack from the rough handling. Pack enough clothes, makeup, and toiletries in your carry-on luggage to get you through three days, just in case your checked luggage gets lost in transit.

SIX
Can't-Miss
Budget Moves

Looking fashionable shouldn't put you in the poorhouse. Some cost-conscious ideas:

1. Fight the impulse to buy something simply because it's on sale, especially if it doesn't fit. Just because it's cheap doesn't mean you need it. How many times have you bought designer shoes for 50 percent off even though they were "a little too tight"?

2. Do a reality check before you step up to the register. If you already own something similar, don't have anything to wear it with, or have an uneasy feeling about the purchase, take it right back to the rack.

3. Use the buddy system by taking a friend along who knows what your budget is and will make sure you stick to it.

4. Shop around to find the best price. Sometimes the savings can be substantial if you comparison shop. Many fashion magazines even have pages that show you how to knock off a designer look on the cheap. Dressing well means more than lining your closet with expensive designer labels. People come up to me all the time, asking, "Isn't that a Divine Devante?" And I say, "Yes, of course." Hey, what they don't know won't hurt them.

5. Leave the charge cards at home. It's easy—and fun—to buy with no cash. But those bills will haunt you.

6. Be patient. Most likely, the item you like will go on sale before the end of the season. Ask the saleswoman in the store for her business card, or ask her to put you on the mailing list, then check in with her periodically about upcoming sales.

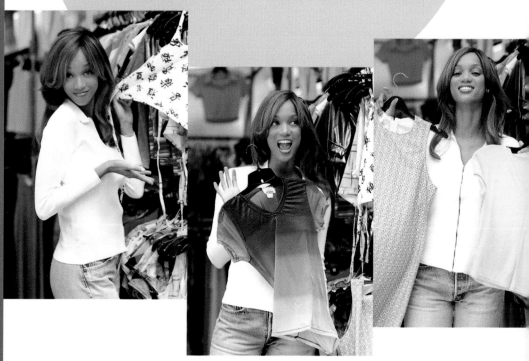

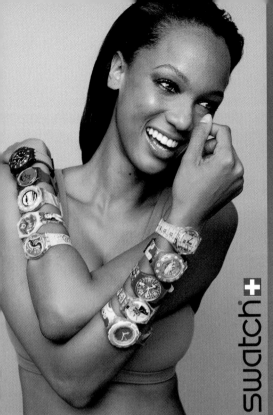

my real jewelry for special occasions. I'm also into inexpensive watches.

I must own a Swatch in every color and design under the sun. They're attractive and fun, as well as durable, which means that they don't get scratched up as easily as those really expensive watches tend to.

I've lost too many pairs of sunglasses to continue to spend good money on them, so I don't. But with bargain shades, you have to be very careful. Your eyes are precious, and bad lenses can cause permanent damage. So you can be thrifty, but beware. You need proper UV protection and clear, non-cloudy, unscratched lenses.

Swatch+

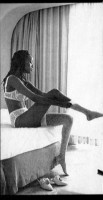

PERFECT IMPOSTERS

I have a bad habit of losing expensive watches, jewelry, and sunglasses. So I've learned to scrimp in those areas. I gave up wearing real jewelry on a day-to-day basis the first time I lost a pair of precious gems at a photo shoot. Now I buy those fake diamond studs made of cut glass. (I don't even buy zircons!) They cost about $8 a pair, so I buy them in bulk and pass them out to my friends like candy. And so what if I lose a pair? I can just reach into my jewelry drawer for a carbon copy. Just be sure when you buy inexpensive jewelry that it's hypoallergenic. (In the past, I've gotten itchy, infected ears from jewelry made from substandard materials.) I save

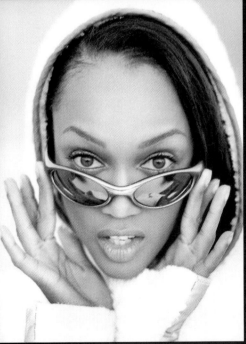

Oldies But Goodies

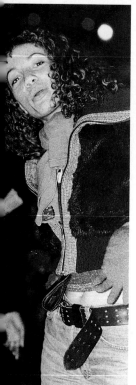

Khefri

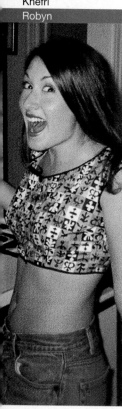

Robyn

My high school friend Khefri was the first person to tell me I should model. From the moment we met, we hit it off big time. I picked up a lot of fashion hints from her, but the coolest tip was shopping in thrift stores. Back then, Khefri knew how to style an outfit from head to toe for $5. Robyn, another good friend of mine, is also a thrift-shop expert. You compliment her on a shirt and she'll proudly tell you that she got it for just a dollar.

To this day, thrift stores are one of my favorite places to shop, especially for vintage jeans. I don't like new jeans—they're too stiff and don't hug me in the right places. I prefer the worn-in kind that hang low like hip huggers, and thrift shops generally have the best selection.

I can spend all afternoon sifting through the racks in search of that one perfect piece. Of course, it takes a lot of patience, because the clothes in many stores can be jumbled together and totally disorganized. So you have to be prepared to examine every article of clothing, because there could be a little gem lurking in the cracks and if you move too fast, you'll miss it.

But take your time and there's no telling what you'll discover, or from which era, from a 1920s flapper dress or a '40s zoot suit to a '50s poodle skirt, a '60s tie-dyed T-shirt, or a pair of '70s designer jeans.

When you're thrifting, it's important to shop at places that clean the clothes before they put them on the racks, otherwise you might come across dirty merchandise on the selling floor. I can't tell you how many times I've fallen in love with something, only to realize one sniff later that it hasn't been cleaned. I usually come prepared to do a whiff test on anything I like. I'm not just testing for funk—I'm also concerned about any mildew, bacteria, or varmits that could be hiding out in the garment. If I detect a musty or unusual odor, I put it back on the rack and move on.

Trying on clothes is even more important where thrifting is concerned because, unlike other stores, you may not be able to return it. Happy hunting!

It doesn't matter what the world says is "hot," "now," or a "must-have." Style isn't about brands or trends or how much money you've spent.

It all comes down to what *you* feel like putting on your body each day.

Clothes speak volumes about you even before you've opened your mouth. The question is, What message do you want to convey?

Who do you want to be today?

A high-powered executive? A big kid? A swanky socialite? A sports jock? A rapper or a rock star? A sultry vamp? A laid-back bohemian?

Fashion allows us to be anything we want to be, without saying a word.

You've probably all seen footage of what goes on behind the scenes at entertainment industry parties –

the music is pumping, the champagne is flowing, and a hazy fog of cigarette smoke hangs in the air.

At first, it seems like it's just one big party, and everybody is joining in. But if that camera would just pan to the back of the room and get a close-up of the girl hanging out in the corner booth, they'd see she was sipping on a ginger ale, not a gin and tonic.

They'd also see that that girl in the back corner booth is usually me.

on a
Flying

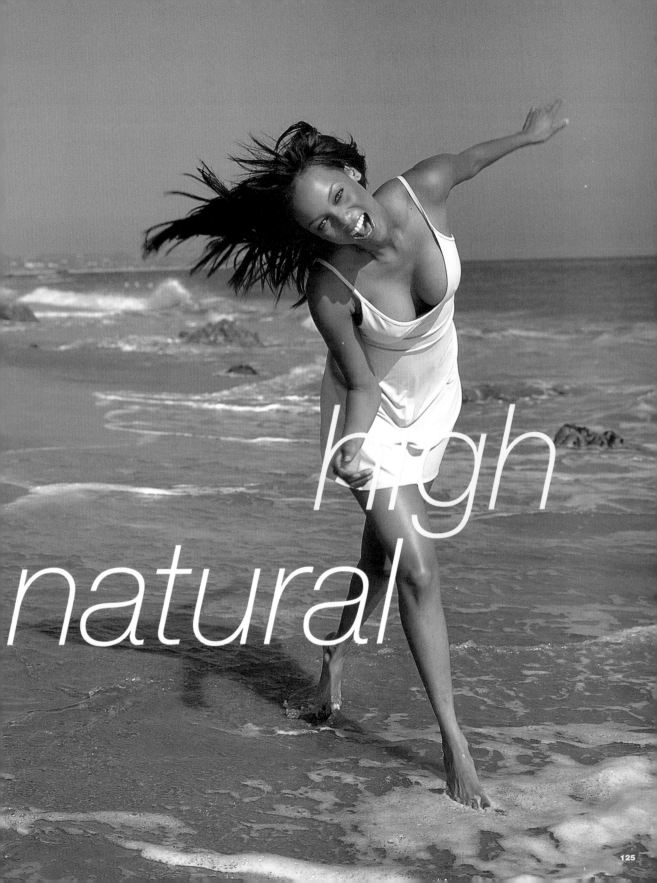

natural

Many people find it hard to believe that
was when I was six years old, or that the
of a wine cooler when I was thirteen. But

A real drag

I remember this experience so vividly. It was a couple of months before my seventh birthday and I was playing hide-and-seek over at a neighbor's house. It was my turn to hide, so I hurried and crouched down behind an end table. I stayed there for what seemed like hours, until I thought it was safe to peek over the top of the table. Instead of spotting my friend, I found myself facing a cigarette burning in an ashtray. Her

incident, I was totally turned off, and to this day, I can't even stand the smell of them.

Cigarettes aren't known as "cancer sticks" for nothing. My grandmother Florine London, who began smoking cigarettes when she was thirteen, died of lung cancer. She was only forty-nine when she was diagnosed. I watched her suffer for nine months. The cancer spread from her lungs to her bones and, finally, to her brain.

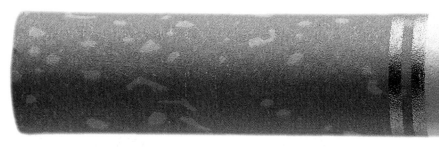

mother, a serious chain-smoker, had left it there.

I guess you could say I let my curiosity get the better of me. I picked up the cigarette and took one *long* drag that filled my entire mouth with smoke. Since I had no experience with smoking, I failed to realize that exhaling was part of the process, and I swallowed the smoke in one great gulp.

I felt hot, scorching pain all the way down my throat and into my lungs. I must have coughed for two days afterward. What an introduction to cigarettes! After that

At that point, my grandmother hardly recognized any of us and would drift in and out of consciousness, all the while in severe pain. At times, she thought she was a little girl again, and would ask my mother to bring her doll to her. And she continually begged my mother to put her out of her misery.

Grandma Florine London

I'd think about her pet name for me, Dee, and burst out in tears because I knew I

he only time a cigarette has touched my lips
most I've ever had to drink was about a quarter
t's the absolute truth.

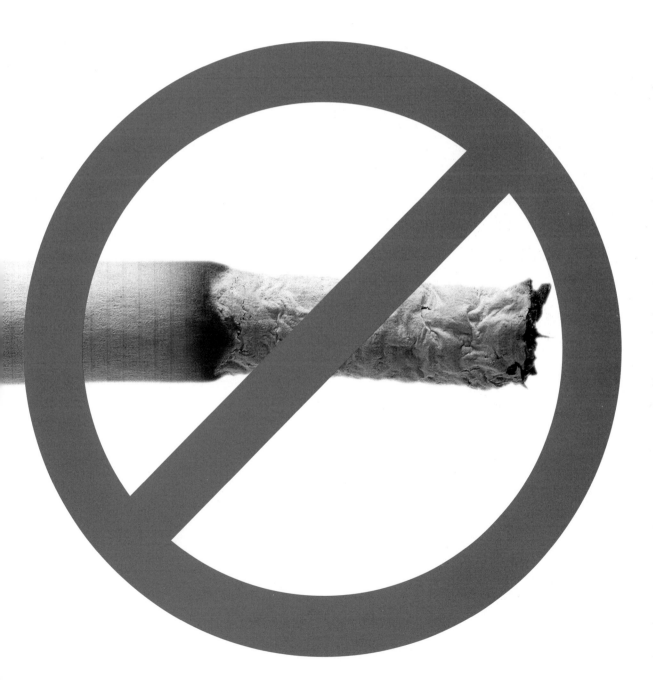

would never hear her call me that again. I felt guilty because there was absolutely nothing I could do to help her.

After months of agony, she died, at the age of fifty. Had she known when she first began smoking that it would cut her life short, I don't think she ever would have started. Back then, there weren't any warnings on cigarette packages that said

SURGEON GENERAL'S WARNING: Smoking Causes Lung Cancer, Heart Disease, Emphysema, And May Complicate Pregnancy.

smoking was addictive and caused cancer. Even now, I think it's hard for many people to believe that those thin white tubes packed with tiny strips of tobacco are lethal. They look harmless enough, especially in advertisements, but of course that's what cigarette manufacturers want us to think.

But the manufacturers aren't entirely to blame. We play a role in the addiction by refusing to believe the statistics that prove smoking is dangerous to our health. I guess it's just human to think that bad things happen only to other people, never to us. We hear so much every day about this food, that drink, the air quality here, and living environments there that are bad for us that we just block it out. But we are not immune.

With my grandmother, I saw up close what habitual smoking can lead to. The images of her last days in the hospital are forever ingrained in my memory. And because of that, I told myself I would not promote smoking.

There's no question I've lost out on a lot of work because of this. I've been asked many times to hold cigarettes in fashion layouts, and I'll admit that I gave in once on a job where the photographer intimidated me. But it made me feel uncomfortable—all I could think about was my grandmother. So now I simply refuse. The last thing I want to do is glamorize the thing that killed a loved one, not to mention millions of other people each year.

When you think about it, what's to glamorize? Cosmetically speaking, cigarettes stain your teeth and your skin, making them look yellow and dingy. They also give you that foul smoker's breath. Have you ever been to a party where lots of people are smoking around you? My lungs feel smoke infused and ache for days afterward. And the smell clings to your clothes—you might as well just take that party outfit straight to the dry cleaners, because the odor won't go away on its own.

The internal effects are just as horrible. I jog with a group of people a couple of times a week and the smokers are forever falling behind. I'm convinced that all that huffing and puffing they do on the running trail is directly related to all that puffing they do on cigarettes. And let's not even talk about the nagging dry cough some smokers can't seem to get rid of after so many years of lighting up. My grandmother coughed and wheezed constantly, but at the time we didn't realize that it was connected to her cigarette smoking.

We're constantly bombarded with information about the ill effects of smoking. It's been broadcast throughout the media, from outdoor billboards to TV public service announcements to the Internet. Politicians from the president on down the line have been some of smoking's strongest and loudest detractors. But I don't think the message can ever be communicated enough. Smoking is *the* leading preventable cause of death among women in the United States. It can lead to lung cancer, emphysema, strokes, and heart disease, as well as severe bronchitis and asthma. The easiest way to avoid these problems is to steer clear of cigarettes altogether.

Kicking **BUTT**

Cigarettes have long been used—and abused—by women as a method of weight control, because smoking curbs the appetite. I recently read a survey in a magazine that said 98 percent of models smoke or have smoked, and I think the connection is more than coincidence. A lot of them are probably lighting up to keep their weight down. But the weight gain that sometimes occurs when a smoker quits is not a given. And the cravings that women feel when they stop smoking can be curbed.

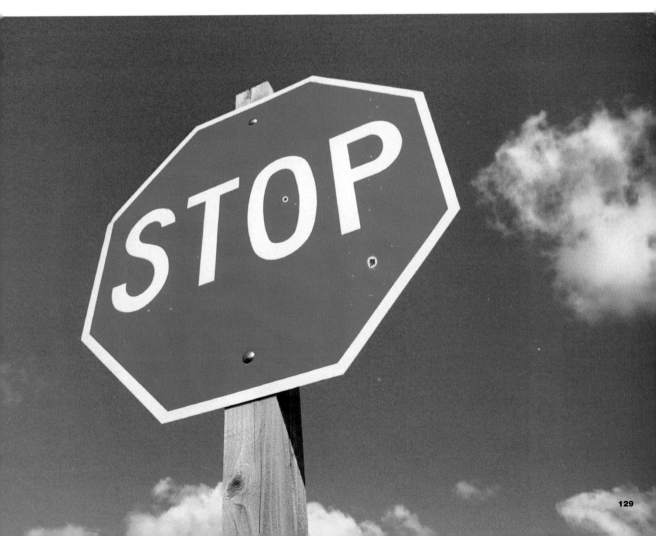

What cigarettes actually do is keep your mouth busy so that you don't look for oral satisfaction elsewhere. But there are many healthier ways to quiet that urge:

Exercise.
Besides the obvious health benefits, you'll be too busy getting buff to worry about feeding your face.

Substitute.
Snack on fresh vegetables and fruit, trail mix, sugarless gum, or even better, down a couple of glasses of water.

Avoid temptation.
Minimize the amount of time you spend in the presence of people who aren't ready to give up their daily dose of nicotine; when they light up, walk away. Sit in the nonsmoking section of a restaurant; if there isn't one, then ask to be seated at a table where you aren't surrounded by smokers. Try not to linger too long in places such as clubs and bars where you'll have a hard time fighting the impulse to puff. Clean out your home of all ashtrays and cigarette packs.

Seek out people who sympathize.
Formalized programs such as Smokenders, where counselors provide advice and encouragement, can wean you from the habit and help you through the rough period. There is a fee involved, but in the overall scheme of things, it probably costs less than it would to maintain your smoking habit. Also, put everyone on notice that you are quitting, and enlist their help in keeping you on the path to a smoke-free existence.

Use products designed to curb addiction.
There are all kinds of nicotine replacement methods on the market, from the patch to nicotine gum, that promise to curb the addiction. The people who seem to do the best with these products are the ones who consult a physician to find the dosage that works for them. It's also important to stay on your routine—if you take dosages haphazardly, the product won't work as effectively.

Reward yourself.
When you've had a good day, good week, good month, give yourself a little pat on the back. Thinking long–term, make plans for the money you'll save from quitting by planning a day of pampering at a spa, or a trip to an exotic island.

Booze**NEWS**

'**ve** been offered alcohol more than any other substance, most likely because it's usually socially acceptable to have a drink. It's rare that I attend a party or other public event where alcohol isn't available, in abundance. In our culture, alcohol and celebration seem to go hand in hand.

Even though I choose not to drink, I don't have a problem if other people want to. What I don't understand is drinking just to get drunk. The time you spend feeling bad–headaches, nausea, vomiting, hangovers–lasts longer than the buzz.

When I was thirteen, I had a friend who seemed to really enjoy drinking herself into a state of unconsciousness. Once when I was hanging out at her house, she pulled out some peach wine coolers and told me to drink one. I took a couple of sips and tried to like it, but the taste disgusted me. The initial peach flavor was fine, but the alcohol aftertaste was too overpowering and ruined any chances of my liking it.

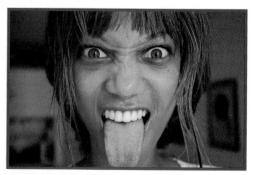

I asked her, "Why are you drinking this when it doesn't even taste good?" She looked like she agreed with me, but said, "Yeah, the taste isn't great, but it makes me feel good." I just let my bottle sit

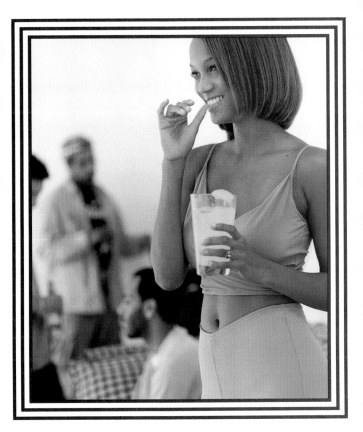

I realized at an early age that drinking was not something I wanted to pursue into adulthood. But it hasn't been easy living with this decision. The outside pressure to drink can be overwhelming, particularly in my profession. People think you are a Goody Two-shoes, or simply uptight. But I often wonder if the ones doing the most scrutinizing secretly wish *they* could refuse a drink without feeling self-conscious.

To tell you the truth, I feel uncomfortable when people are intoxicated around me. Since I've never experienced this, I don't know what's going on in their heads—and that scares me.

Don't get me wrong. Even though I don't indulge, I'm perfectly fine with others having a drink. I just think it's wise to exercise some moderation. Unfortunately, some people don't know when to stop.

there and watched her while she finished off two more. Then she downed the rest of mine, threw up her lunch, and passed out beside me.

Ever since then, I find it easy to pass up a drink, though it sure seems to make other people feel uneasy. It was most obvious when I first started modeling. Whenever I refused a drink, I would get strange looks, as if to say, "Who is she trying to impress?" But now, after running into the same people over and over in all kinds of social settings, they're getting used to passing me a virgin piña colada instead of one spiked with rum. People often tell me they want to be the first ones to see me drunk, and my response is always the same: "It's not going to happen."

I had a friend in high school whose personality changed when she drank. She took it to the extreme—falling down, passing out on the lawn, vomiting—the whole nine yards. But she was my friend, so I tried to help her in the best way I could.

I even got in trouble with the police one time because of her. We were headed to a party in separate cars, and I guess she decided that she was going to start partying on the way there. She had one hand on the steering wheel and the other wrapped around a beer bottle. Her car was doing so much swerving and weaving that it was obvious to me, and probably to anyone else who saw her, that there was a problem. We turned onto a street that was lined with police cars, and I was sure the police would arrest her if she was spotted. So I purposely made a left-hand turn from the right lane so that the police would be distracted from her and follow me. The police took the bait, pulled me over, and gave me a ticket.

DRINK DRIVE DIE

I thought I was defusing the situation, but now I know that the best way to have helped her would have been to let her get caught. She would have been forced to take responsibility for her actions, and maybe the experience would have been so frightening that she would have learned from it. Instead, I placed myself in a situation that put my safety in danger. Luckily, the only thing that was damaged was my driving record.

I understand why drinking can be appealing, especially when times get tough. I've been hurt, disappointed, angry, and frustrated—all reasons I might have for seeking comfort from a bottle—and I can see how alcohol might dull my pain. But it's a temporary fix. The problem will still be there long after the last traces of intoxication have worn off.

I'm lucky enough to have friends and family to turn to during the tough times. They help me to work through the pain, so there's no need to turn to booze in order to feel better. The support they give me lasts longer than a drink ever could.

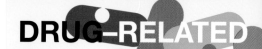

DRUG-RELATED

Stories about drug use in the modeling world seem to resurface every couple of years, and these last few have been no different. Some claim it's the seventies all over again, with people passing heroin needles and cocaine around on sterling-silver platters, and slipping in and out of drug-treatment centers. The Oval Office even got involved last year when the president publicly denounced the "heroin chic" look (super-skinny girls who looked as if they were under the influence of the drug) used in fashion magazine spreads and advertising.

I can honestly tell you that I've never been offered drugs on a job. But the simple fact is that drugs are everywhere, in all walks of life, not just the fashion, film, and music industries. You don't have to see pushers dealing on a street corner to know that they exist. Dealers are stalking the corporate corridors of big business and hiding behind the polished mahogany doors of million-dollar homes. The idea that the entertainment industry and inner-city ghettos are the only drug havens is a total fiction.

When I was growing up, I never had the desire to experiment with drugs, and the same went for most of the people I hung out with. But I sure was shocked when I found out how many of my classmates did.

The funny thing is, our school had representatives from antidrug organizations coming in constantly to give speeches. We would politely sit in these assemblies and patiently listen while the police officers and health care workers told us to "Just say no." Actually what I think they should have been saying was "Just stop doing it." There were too many students who were already either experimenting with or addicted to drugs to talk to us as if we were totally oblivious.

I think the reinforcement I received at home is what *really* kept me from experimenting with drugs. Ma didn't sit me down and give me a big speech about the dangers involved. She'd just share stories about the friends she grew up with who had gotten into drugs and how it had ruined their lives. Then she'd tell me about getting a natural high.

Ma lived through the whole hippie culture when most young people thought it was cool to do drugs. Her friends would call her a square and a prude for not joining in, but she never gave in to the peer pressure. In fact, she was still the life of the party, without any artificial stimulants influencing her. She danced herself into a sweat for hours and laughed with such gusto that people would say, "Give me some of what she's on!" But she wasn't on anything—it was all 100 percent pure and natural energy.

She must have passed on some of those same traits to me, because I've been known to be just as uninhibited. Like my mom, I'm so pumped up when I'm out with my friends that people think I'm actually on something too! But I tell them, "I'm flying on a natural high." Most people don't get it.

It may sound clichéd, but I get high on life. The best way I can describe it is to say that it's like the feeling you get when you're with a bunch of your friends and you start joking around, and then somebody else says something really funny and you can't stop laughing. Your sides start to hurt, and by now you're laughing so hard you think you're going to lose control of your bladder, but you manage to pull yourself together. Then as soon as you regain your composure, somebody else says something even more hilarious and there you are, racing to the rest room before you pee on yourself. I'm talking about spontaneous fun, plain and simple!

I don't doubt that drugs make people feel good. If they didn't, there wouldn't be so many people willing to give up everything—family, friends, job, personal possessions—to get that next high. The pull is so seductive that you either can't fight it or won't even try.

With some drugs, after the first hit, you're hooked. Some say it's like floating on a cloud without a care in the world. But like clouds, the feeling eventually disappears into thin air and then you're left with nothing to hold on to. I always remind myself: If something feels too good to be true, it probably is.

ill pills

In movies and on television shows, we've all seen the old comedy routine about a man slipping something into a woman's drink so that he can take advantage of her. Unfortunately, the sad truth is that in recent times, this plot line has become a very real problem across the country. And it's nothing to laugh at.

A drug called Rohypnol, also known as "roofies," "ruffies," "rope," or "la roche," has earned a reputation as the "date-rape drug." The drug is illegal in the United States, yet it is being used to lower women's inhibitions, everywhere from high school house parties to bars and nightclubs, and even on dates.

Rohypnol is a heavy-duty sedative. In fact, it's said to be ten times stronger than Valium. When combined with alcohol, it dramatically increases the effects of drunkenness. You might not be able to talk in complete sentences or take two steps without stumbling. Its worst effect is that you may not know where you are or remember how you got there.

"Roofies" usually have no odor and no taste, so it's impossible to tell if they've been added to your drink. Nationwide, there are a number of cases where women have been sexually assaulted while under the effects of this drug. By the time a woman who has been drugged with Rohypnol realizes that something has gone wrong, it's usually too late. Many do not press charges because they can't recall any details. So BE CAREFUL! Some places to start:

Refuse to be catered to. I mean this in a good way. If a guy offers to get a drink for you at a party, politely turn down his offer and get it yourself. I always do this because I'm afraid someone might try to spike my drink.

Don't worry about wasting it. If you put down a drink to go to the dance floor or take a trip to the rest room, don't go back to that drink. Once it's out of your line of vision, someone might slip something into it. Either keep the drink with you, or, if you've put it down, just buy a new one. The short-term expense is worth it if it spares you some grief in the long run.

Five Feel-Good
MOOD BOOSTERS

Whenever life gets you down, you don't have to drown your sorrows in alcohol, pop some pills, or try to puff your troubles away. A few vice-free alternatives:

Call a good friend. Talk to someone who always lifts your spirits and invite her (or him!) over, or go visit her so you don't feel alone.

Spoil yourself. Take some time to give yourself some special treatment, like a long, hot bubble bath. Light some candles and play some soothing music. Let the peace and quiet sink in.

Have a good laugh. Rent a funny movie or watch a sitcom that keeps you in stitches.

Get in the spirit. For some people, prayer can be a tremendous mood lifter. Meditation or simply stealing some quiet time to be alone with your thoughts can also put things in perspective.

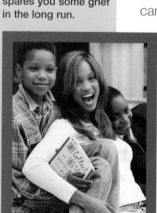

Volunteer. It's hard to be self-destructive when you're busy helping others. The good feeling you get from giving of yourself is its own reward.

We all have the strength within us to sidestep substance abuse. With some people, it seems to have kicked in at birth. Others are lucky enough to have support systems like parents, friends, and partners who help bring that strength to the surface. If, for the moment, you don't have the advantage of either, don't give up.

There are many organizations with people who care and are ready to extend a helping hand.

Just because I play an angel on TV doesn't mean I am perfect.

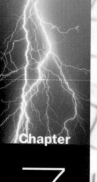

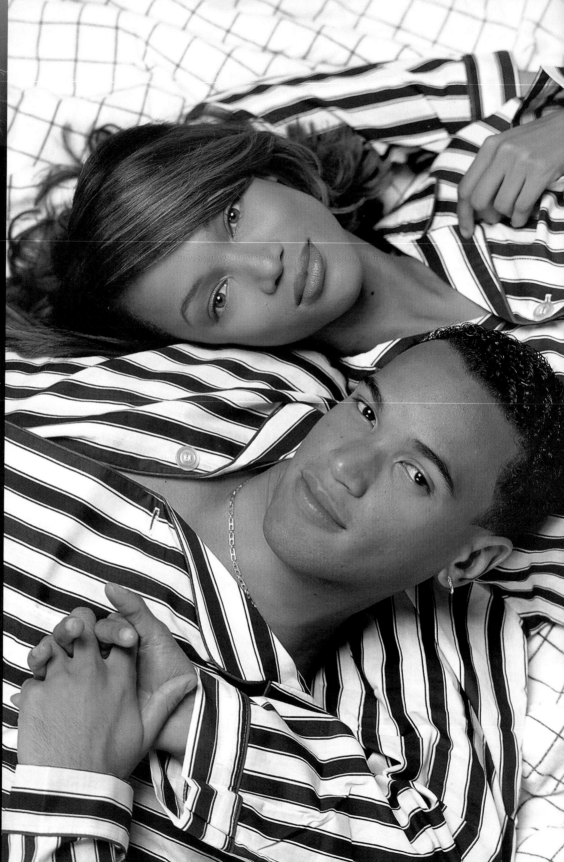

All of the men depicted in this chapter are models. The quoted statements were not necessarily made by the individuals pictured.

Whenever I get into long conversations with my buddies, the discussion inevitably works its way around to men. We talk about who's got a man, and who doesn't (usually me), who's man is tripping, and who just kicked her man to the curb. Occasionally I'll offer up a story of my own to get some insight.

Lord knows I've had my share of love WOES.

I don't know how many of you have said the words "I love you," but I think I've uttered them more than once too often. When the relationship is going strong, you're all into it, like,

"Oh, my God.
I can't live without him."

But then, when the relationship ends, the thought of him makes you want to puke. So then you begin to wonder, Was that love? Real, true, honest-to-goodness love?

I know I've had crushes, and I've been crushed. Those relationships were more about being in love with the romantic and idealized image of that person—dreaming big dreams and fantasizing. But then I'd get to know the guy better, and the bubble would completely burst.

Fortunately, I've been lucky enough to experience the warm, fuzzy, wonderful side of love too. The feeling I got when I was truly in love with someone was completely different from the feeling I got from a crush.

There was friendship
as well as romantic love.

It was easy to be with him, comfortable, secure. I didn't try to make him over into some perfect image I'd built up in my mind. I had my eyes wide open and could see him for who he really was, and was truly happy with what I saw. It's a feeling I've had only once so far, and I hope that one day I'll again be fortunate enough to feel that way about someone.

From that experience, I know how beautiful love can be, and how complex, especially when "doin' the nasty" enters the picture. One day you're floating on air, the next day totally confused. I think everyone who has been in a relationship has felt that way at some point. And when I talk to my friends, it just confirms that I'm not alone. We learn so much from other people's experiences–especially when it comes to sex and romance. It helps to know that I'm not the only one going through such drama.

That's why, for this chapter, I consulted a range of young women of diverse ethnicities, occupations, and ages, from women in their teens to women in their twenties, and asked them to share some of their relationship stories. And so, I apologize to anyone who turned to this chapter to hear all about what *I* do behind closed doors.

I'll tell some… but not all.

I'm proud to say I shot these pics myself.

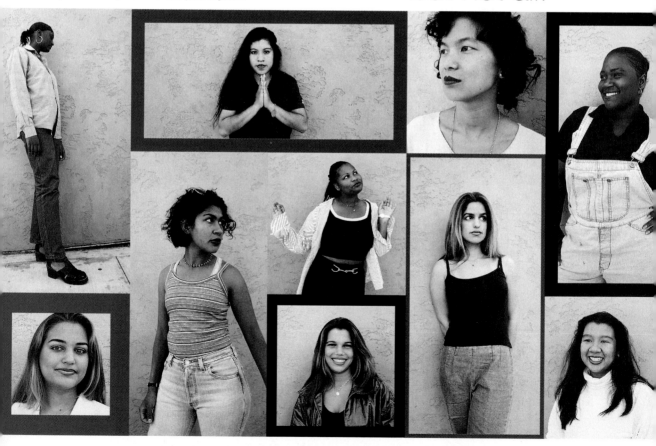

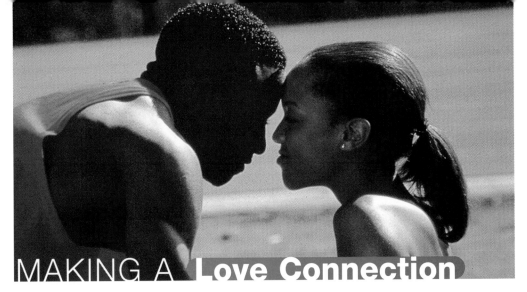

MAKING A Love Connection

Whenever I don't have a steady boyfriend, my buddies try to hook me up with someone. A lot of times I'll just say I'm not interested right now, but every once in a while I'll cave in. They haven't all been great experiences, and they *definitely* haven't all swept me off my feet. But they have all been useful because they've helped me to figure out what I do and don't like, what I'll deal with, and what I won't stand for.

If I could describe my ideal date, I would say it would start out with a guy who picks me up on time. We'd go out to a nice restaurant where we would have a tasty meal and talk for hours. I'd offer to split the tab, and he wouldn't have a problem with it. And he'd treat me like a lady—opening the car door, pulling out my chair for me, all of those old-fashioned things. We'd have a great conversation with no sexual innuendo. We'd laugh and joke so much that it wouldn't feel like we were on a date at all.

Although I've come close, I haven't had that perfect date yet. But I've sure had my share of disasters.

There was a guy in my neighborhood I'd had my eye on for months, so a few days after my sixteenth birthday, I mustered up the nerve to ask him out. His name was Derek, and he was on the local hockey team. He was an older man: nineteen, a freshman in college, and gorgeous. Of course I thought I was *all that* for going out with a superfine college man.

He took me to see *The Little Mermaid*, which sounds pretty innocent, right? But ten minutes into the movie, he started talking about how fine the mermaid was and what a great body she had. In my mind, I was thinking,

"Hello—reality check! She's a cartoon!"

At the time, I was skinny and underdeveloped so I started to feel a little inadequate. I felt that he was comparing *me* to the *mermaid*! By the time we left, I was fuming. Believe it or not, I went out with him again…and again…and again. In fact, we dated, on and off, for two years. But when we went to the movies to see *Beauty and the*

Beast and he started going on and on about how sexy Belle was, then I knew it was time to move on.

Once, on another date, I told the guy I would pick him up at his house. I expected him to be ready, but when I arrived, he hadn't even showered yet! What was worse was 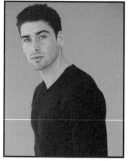 that he didn't even seem to care. After he let me inside, he told me I could wait in the living room with six of his buddies. They were really rowdy–hooting and hollering–and they kept telling me how lucky I was to be going out with their friend. I felt a sudden urge to get away from them, so I decided to wait in the car. It's lucky that I had the radio to distract me because I must have sat outside for about forty-five minutes while "Mr. Popular" primped and preened.

I've been on dates with guys who did nothing but talk about their résumés and how many famous Hollywood actresses they'd "done," and I've been out to dinner with someone who spent the entire time looking at himself in the mirrored wall behind me.

But even after these less than successful experiences, I'm still willing to put myself out there and date because I'm not about to let a few trifling guys spoil it for me. You know, it's like they say, "You've got to kiss a lot of frogs before you find a prince."

Lately it seems like I constantly get the court jester.
But I figure I'll eventually hit on royalty.

Whatta Man, Whatta Man, Whatta Man

Ask any two women what they like in a man and the answers are bound to be as broad as their personalities and interests. I soon found that out when I asked the girls in our discussion group to tell what turns them on:

TurnONS

"Tall, chocolatey, bowlegged men, like Hill Grant."

"You mean **GRANT HILL**."

"Whatever, all I know is that he's fine."

"Smart, nerdy types–the kind you find in band or study hall."

"New York guys with attitude, and bald, like LL Cool J."

"Someone with high standards of hygiene, like men who get manicures."

"Brad Pitt–those eyes, those lips!"

"Shoes are important; you can be fine, but if your shoes are raggedy, that's a turnoff."

"Jimmy Smits is one of the sexiest men on the planet. ¡Ay, papi!"

TurnOFFS

"A boring personality."

"Laziness."

"Bad breath."

"I once went out with a guy who didn't want to do anything but lay around and drink tea. There's more to life than tea!"

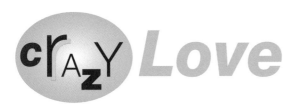

crazy Love

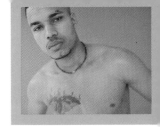

Everybody's got a story about the loony things they've done for love. Just when I think I've heard it all, someone tells me something more outrageous. Of course to them, at the time, their actions probably didn't seem that crazed. These girls from our group discussion say they can laugh about it now, but back then…

Elaine: *One time my boyfriend got kicked out of his house, so I told him he could sleep over at my house–on the porch. I didn't tell my parents because I thought he'd be gone before they woke up. What I didn't know was that he'd brought five of his friends along. The next morning, when my father went outside to get the paper, he tripped right over my boyfriend. I got in so much trouble.*

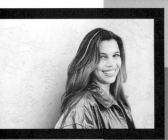

Wendy: *If I suspect a guy is cheating on me, I have to find out for sure. I've done it all–spying on him, snooping through his things. I've even gotten hold of his voice-mail code and checked his messages.*

Diane: *I was so convinced my boyfriend was seeing someone else that I went to his job and confronted him. I was like a madwoman–yelling, screaming, throwing things. I went crazy. They had to call building security on me!*

Tyra: *When I was fourteen I started dating this older guy (he was eighteen) I'd met at a New Edition/Bobby Brown/Al B. Sure concert. I lied about my age and we started dating, but when my parents found out how old he was, they wouldn't let me see him anymore. Of course, that made me want to see him even more, so I'd sneak behind their backs. One time I told them that I was meeting my friends at the mall when I was actually supposed to meet him. They told me it was too late at night to go out, so instead I sat in my bedroom pouting, listening to the radio. A call-in contest came on, and I got through and actually won. When the DJ came on, he asked me what I was doing home alone on a Friday night. I told him how I was supposed to meet this guy at the mall, but couldn't, and how mad I was. The next thing I knew, my stepfather was knocking on my bedroom door. He had been listening to the radio! I got in so much trouble–no phone privileges, no going out, nothing!*

I think about some of the lengths I've gone to and ask myself, Was it really worth it? Some of it I chalk up to just being young and crazy. But sometimes there's more to it than that. As we talked about it in the discussion group, some of the girls said that women go to these lengths because we get more

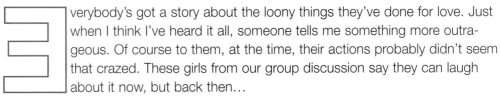

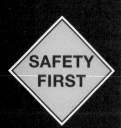
Getting to know someone takes time. So whenever you're going out with someone for the first time or the first few times, I think it's important to take a few precautions until you know the person a little better. A few safeguards:

Let somebody else know where you're going, like a parent, another close relative, or a friend. Also tell them when you expect to be back.

Organize a group outing that involves several couples. Not only is it safer, but it takes some of the pressure off you if you get a sudden case of bashfulness.

Meet during the day in a place that's public, such as a restaurant or museum. It may not be intimate, but your date will be less likely to try something unacceptable. Many times people associate nighttime with sexual activity.

Have money of your own in case something goes wrong. I was taught to always carry "mad cash" so that I would be able to catch a cab if anything got out of hand. It's a habit I still have.

emotionally involved than men, and we put our feelings first, which gets us into trouble. There's a lot of truth to that, but I also think that sometimes we become so desperate to have a boyfriend that we'll do anything—and put up with everything—to keep him. I think most of us eventually wise up and decide that those kind of men aren't worth all the drama they put us through, especially when there are so many others out there who won't give us grief. Then we begin to look for the kinds of relationships that fulfill us and give us what we need. Of course, we have to know what we want, then go for it. No compromises! Because he's out there. We just have to be patient.

Too CLOSE For COMFORT

Most of the girls I talk to say couples are supposed to share everything, but at least one girl I talked to, Karen, fourteen, didn't agree. "I used to think that I wanted a boyfriend who went to my high school," she said, "but then I realized we probably wouldn't have anything to talk about because we'd know everything about each other already. We'd eat lunch together, walk down the halls together. All the time. Every day. Yuck!"

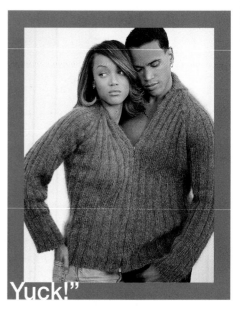

No matter how close two people are, there are times when each person needs some time alone. When a couple spends all their time together, they sometimes end up sacrificing some parts of their lives that make them well-rounded individuals.

I've done that in relationships—put other things on hold to focus all of my attention on the relationship. And it's not healthy. Not too long ago I was dating a guy steadily, and before I knew it I became a real slug. Before we started going out, I was so active—hanging out with my friends, going to the movies, going out to eat. But once I started dating him, I dropped everything (I would even turn down important modeling jobs) and just laid around the house all day waiting for him to call. I had no other interests, and I think that was stifling for him because I was all up under the guy. After a few months, he broke up with me. I think he just got bored.

That experience taught me a valuable lesson. The time we spend apart can be just as important as the time we spend together, because it allows us to grow in ways that bring more to the relationship. Having other close friendships outside the relationship prevents us from putting too much pressure on our partner to be our all and all. **So give him some space—and demand your own.**

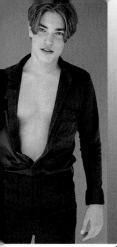

Friends & Lovers

Have you ever been tempted to take a platonic friendship to a romantic level? In some ways, it makes a lot of sense. When you date a close friend, you don't have to put up a front, because he knew you when, so it cuts down on a lot of the time you'd spend feeling out the other person. This is a person who knows the good, the bad, and the ugly about you. He's seen that side that you may not let a stranger see because you're trying to make a good impression. You can be you.

Ultimately, I think we all want to feel comfortable enough in a relationship to be ourselves and be accepted, and being friends is a good place to start. But there's also a gray area. I've never dated someone who was a buddy first, and I think it's because I don't want to lose the friendship if things don't work out. (Well, actually, I'm not really attracted to any of my guy friends–sorry, guys.) What if we break up? Will the relationship be as good as it was before? That's why I'd think before making that move; you have to figure out if this is destiny or just your curiosity getting the better of you. A good man is hard to find, but a good friend is harder to find. Lots of times, boyfriends go in and out of your life, but good friends stay around forever. If you can combine friendship and love without losing either, then it's the best of both worlds!

Heartbreak Hotel

Some people think every guy out there desperately wants to date models, but there are *plenty* of them who don't. Since I first started dating, I've had only three boyfriends, and all of them left me heartbroken and crying on my mother's shoulder. One of them, while not the most serious relationship I've ever had, still really tore me apart. When we broke up, I went into a deep depression. I couldn't eat much for weeks, and wound up losing fifteen pounds. People noticed the change outside, but no one knew what was going on inside. I went to an industry party and everyone was complimenting me on how thin I was and how great I looked. But I thought I looked sick, underweight, and miserable.

Thank God for Ma! She kept me from driving over to the guy's house and begging and pleading for an answer to the question of why he broke up with me. The heartache lasted about three months (but the food thing lasted only three weeks–I love food too much to give that up).

Like they say in the song, breaking up *is* hard to do. When a relationship is over, you must learn to let it go. Probably the worst thing you could do would be to get serious about someone else right away. I know that the temptation to rush into a new relationship is strong (you know what I'm talking about–the rebound boyfriend), but it's definitely not fair to the new person you're seeing.

Now, whenever I start feeling sorry for myself when my heart's been broken, I try to take all that energy I would have wasted moaning and crying, and direct it into something positive. I've come away with some great hobbies because of this. After that last breakup, I took up painting pottery. Not only did it take my mind off my troubles, but now I have all of these personal creations, from ceramic bowls to salt and pepper shakers, that I made to decorate my home and those of my close friends. But now my buddies say, ***"Enough pottery, Tyra."*** The next time my heart is broken, I've got to find a new hobby.

> **WEAK PICK-UP LINE #1:**
>
> A guy came up to me in the mall once and handed me his card, saying, "If you ever need a doctor, give me a call." He was a gynecologist!

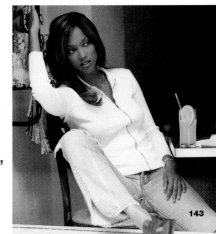

143

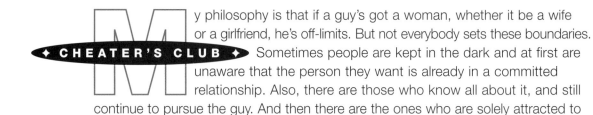

My philosophy is that if a guy's got a woman, whether it be a wife or a girlfriend, he's off-limits. But not everybody sets these boundaries. Sometimes people are kept in the dark and at first are unaware that the person they want is already in a committed relationship. Also, there are those who know all about it, and still continue to pursue the guy. And then there are the ones who are solely attracted to men who are taken. Here are some views from different sides of the love triangle:

Diane: *I had a friend with a boyfriend who put the "d" in dog. He was horrible, just disgusting, and he cheated on her right in front of her face. I asked her what was wrong with her, that she would put up with that. All she said was, "He may be cheating with all these women, but he comes home to me at night."*

Cheryl: *I've been cheated on before, and I know how that hurts. But I've gone out with a married man. I didn't care because I didn't know his wife.*

Ramona: *I was seeing my brother's friend, who was married. I even knew his wife, but I didn't care. She wasn't pretty, anyway. He left her and was with me for two years. Then he left me for someone else.*

Cheryl: *Guys are gonna be guys. If he likes you, so what if he's taken? Go for it!*

Ramona: *I'll never do it again.*

Tyra: *I've had guys try to put one over on me. This one guy told me that he had a girl, but said, "We're on the outs," and I believed him. Luckily for me, I got out before I got too deeply involved.*

Teresa: *I wouldn't want anyone who had someone else. That would be selling myself short. I'd want him thinking about me at night. Not me and Suzy.*

Erica: *Don't you want to be able to call his house and not worry about his wife or girl answering the phone?*

Cheryl: *PAGE HIM!*

Supermodel or not, I have been cheated on. I guess, for some men, there will always be something new and more exciting around the corner. But I understand where Cheryl is coming from. She's dealing with the hurt and anger of having been cheated on. And once that happens, it can desensitize you. You may decide that what's good for him is good for you too as a way of getting some revenge. But the answer is not retaliation: Two wrongs don't make a right.

As women, we should learn from our own experiences and look out for each other so that what has happened and hurt us doesn't happen to someone else and cause them the same pain. There's so much talk about the man shortage that we think we have to share a man. But it's important to think about the other innocent people you could be hurting. You may not know the other woman, but try to remember that she is a human being with feelings and emotions just like yours.

The truth is, there are plenty of available men out there who don't have girlfriends or wives. So leave that involved man alone. Because if he's cheating *with* you, you better believe that later he'll be cheating *on* you.

But the cheating thing goes both ways. If you feel like cheating on your mate, then it's best to get out of the relationship. Holding off on hurting him doesn't help, it just prolongs the agony. If you are honest and up-front, then you won't wind up hurting that person's feelings (or not that badly).

I've always been a one-man woman. Once I agree to see that one person and no one else, I stick with it. Just like anything else in life, I strongly believe that we have to keep our commitments.

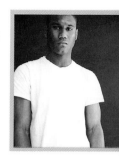

(dreams)

Cinderella

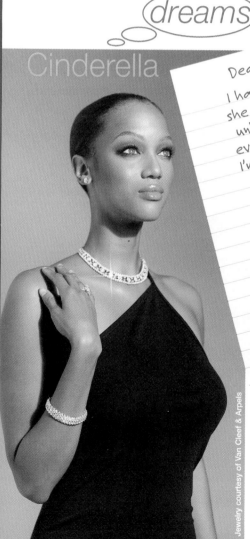

Jewelry courtesy of Van Cleef & Arpels

March 12, 1994

Dear Diary,

I have a friend who swears up and down that she is not a gold digger. But she won't date a guy unless he's rich and famous, in that order. She even quotes guys' salaries to me over the phone. I'm sorry, but in my opinion, "Miss Thing" is definitely **digging for gold.**

People always say to me, "Tyra, when you want to stop modeling, just marry a rich man so he can take care of you. And definitely get married in California, because if you ever get a divorce, you'll get half."

I have a whole lot of friends who live by that rule. One of them, Lisa, goes out with an up-and-coming media mogul. He beats her and cheats on her, and she knows all about his other women. But when I asked her why she wouldn't leave him, she said, "What happens if I leave him and he becomes the next mega-millionaire?" I didn't say anything, but I should have said, "What could happen is that you could leave him, and he could become the next mega-millionaire, and you could find someone who doesn't beat you or cheat on you. Or you could stay with him and just accept the cheating and beating, and hope that he doesn't go too far one day and kill you. But, hey, at least 'd have all that money. ♡T

145

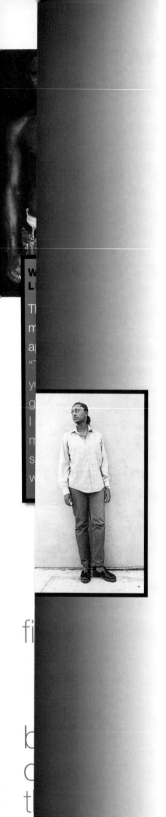

Tyra: *In the beginning it might be attractive to have someone watching over you, but then you realize that that person is just insecure and needs to control you.*

Erica: *That is so true. My first girlfriend was thirty years old. I was in the twelfth grade at the time. The first four months were good. But then she started to get jealous of my friends and told me I couldn't be friends with them anymore. She told me to quit my job, and that she would support me, so I quit. She even took my driving test for me. Once, when we were out at a club, another girl asked me to dance, so I asked my girlfriend if it was okay. I felt like she owned me so I asked permission. She let me dance with her, but then later on she got drunk and grabbed me by the arm and forced me to leave the club. While we were driving in the car, she just kept yelling at me, "You know how jealous I get!" And then she punched the window with her hand, so hard that the windshield shattered. Then she hit me in the eye, and my eye got big and swollen. I tried to jump out of the car, but we were moving about seventy-five miles an hour and I couldn't get away. She lost control of the car and we hit the freeway divider. When her airbag opened up, I ran out of the car and waved down cars until some- one stopped to help me.*

Tyra: *So how did the relationship end?*

Erica: *I didn't want to leave her. But she started beating me every weekend. Finally, I moved out and got my own apartment. That didn't stop her. One day I was on the phone with a friend saying I was going to leave her for good. The next thing I know, my girlfriend is in my house, saying, "Oh, you're gonna leave me, huh?" She snatched the phone out of my hand, pulled the phone cord out of the socket, and started to beat me. The apartment manager heard me screaming and tried to help, but my girlfriend was so strong he couldn't pull her off me. I got hold of a kitchen knife and started stabbing her. I stabbed her seven times. She went to the hospital, and I got arrested, but the charges were later dropped because it was self-defense. To this day, she still wants to be with me.*

All of the behaviors these women describe fit the cycle of abuse that is typical of these kinds of relationships. After a big blowup, the abuser tries to make amends and everything will be cool for a while, until the abuse starts up all over again. Many times the victim will blame herself for what has happened to her; other times people will say she brought it on herself.

I have a friend who sought help from her pastor, who had seen her come to church with bruises and scars. He told her that her husband was probably just having a bad time, so she should try harder to be a good wife. The pastor also told her that whatever she did, she was not to leave her husband, because divorce was a sin. She eventually left anyway, six years later and after losing her hearing in one ear.

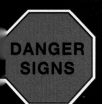

No matter how someone tries to explain his or her behavior away, there is no excuse for abuse. Abusers act this way to assert control and gain power over the victims. Maybe they witnessed this kind of behavior in their own homes growing up and learned it there, or perhaps they were abused as children or had psychological problems that went undiagnosed and untreated. But their reasoning does not have to be your fate.

Once you decide you're ready to leave, you can make it happen. But you've got to have a plan. This is something very difficult to overcome alone, so you must get help. Tell someone. Do not be embarrassed; you did nothing wrong. You do not deserve this treatment. You may have feelings of indecision and then regret, wondering whether you've done the right thing. But in time these feelings will fade. You must realize that the situation will not get better; it will only worsen. A push becomes a shove. A shove becomes a slap. A slap becomes a punch. A punch becomes a beating. I firmly believe that my two friends would not be here today if they had not taken those first steps to make new lives for themselves. This is the kind of situation in which it pays to put yourself first. It could save your life.

RAPE Facts vs. Fiction

There are all kinds of misconceptions surrounding the subject of rape, and the debate over date rape has only made it more controversial. Too often, women are accused of either making the whole thing up, putting themselves in compromising positions that lead others to believe they are willing to have have sex, or dressing in a way that says they are promiscuous.

The facts are that women do not choose to be raped, they are forced. The rapist is interested in sexual domination at all costs, and may even believe that old "no-means-yes" school of thought. Brute force doesn't even necessarily have to be a factor. We've all heard the stories about the woman who went to a frat party, had one drink too many, and hours later woke up half dressed in somebody's room. Whatever the circumstances, if a woman has sex without giving her consent, it's rape. And sex isn't the rapist's objective – aggression is.

What scares me is how skeptical we've all become about the reality of rape. I've heard one too many people say that "the woman should have known better." Here are stories from girls in our discussion group. It is surprising how many of them had experienced, or knew someone who had experienced, being raped:

Delia: *My cousin was raped by a family member. She told my aunt about it, but no one believed her. Now she doesn't talk about it to anyone.*

Tyra: *That's very common – family members trying to keep their skeletons in the closet.*

Stephanie: *I had a friend who was raped by my cousin's boyfriend. She told the family, and they all went over and shot up his house! I have one cousin serving time* *in prison now because he got caught at the scene shooting up the house. My friend used to be happy and perky, but now she's sad all the time. She doesn't even comb her hair. She's in a constant state of depression and refuses to talk to anyone or get help.*

Diane: *Whenever I get into deep conversations with other girls, I constantly hear them confessing to me that they've been raped. They're always afraid to tell some-body, especially if it's someone in the family who did it. They're, like, "Oh, Mama's gonna be mad if I tell on Uncle, or if I tell on Daddy." I've only heard one story where the mom supported the girl. Her mom wound up putting her own brother in jail.*

Audrey: *I was raped. I met this guy and every time he would come to pick me up, he never wanted to come in and meet my mom. I thought it was strange, but I just ignored it. One day we were supposed to go to the movies, but we didn't. We ended up back at his house. He raped me. Afterward, I thought I was pregnant. He gave me chlamydia. It was so hard for me because I didn't tell anyone, not even my best friend, for a year. When we would go out with guys I always had to have her there with me but she never knew why. But she had to be there. I never went out without her. I didn't want to be touched by a man and was uncomfortable when one looked at me. And the pain and hurt didn't stop until I sat down and told my best friend. My advice is that when you go out with a man, you have to really know and trust him. This man put me in a situation where I was helpless. He gave me a disease, and to this day I don't know if I can have kids because I might be sterile. I can't tell my mom. Eventually I guess one day I will tell her. But she always warned me about how to be safe and it still happened to me. I feel like I didn't listen to her.*

> Only 26 percent of all rapes or attempted rapes are reported to law enforcement officials.

Tyra: *Oh, no, Audrey. You listened to your mom. This guy could have had a parent he didn't listen to. So it wasn't your fault. This could have happened to every single one of us in this room.*

Audrey said that you have to know someone before you go out with him in order to tell if he is violent. But a guy who rapes doesn't always show the signs of a potential aggressor. Sometimes the warning signs come only moments before the attack. There is no typical profile for who is and isn't a rapist. A 1994 study conducted by the U.S. Department of Justice found that about 28 percent of rape victims are raped by husbands or boyfriends, 35 percent by acquaintances, and 5 percent by relatives. The same study revealed that only 26 percent of all rapes or attempted rapes are reported to law enforcement officials.

More victims need to come forward. And that will only happen when we create an environment in which women feel they can be heard and believed, from the moment they make that call to the police, to the people they encounter at the hospital, to the family and friends who can help with the healing process.

It also takes courage on the victim's part. Reporting a rape is almost like reliving the act all over again. As much as you want to forget about it, you've got to tell someone, because the attacker must be stopped before he rapes again. **If you are raped, there are a few things you should do:**

Get to the hospital emergency room immediately. Do not clean up first; you will be washing away valuable evidence. The examination will be difficult—the doctors will need to do a pelvic exam as well as survey your external injuries, if any. You may be given treatments for STDs or "morning-after" pills if you are afraid that you might become pregnant.

Talk to somebody about it. After the police have questioned you, seek out support: a parent, a friend, someone on the hospital staff (a rape counselor or psychiatrist may be on hand), or ask for a referral to a support group. It's important to share your feelings. Keeping them inside will only magnify the pain.

Don't expect to feel like yourself for a while. Rape is a life-altering experience, but it doesn't have to be debilitating. There are professionals who can help you through the emotional swings. You don't have go through this alone.

Dear Diary,

To Do It or Not to Do It

July 7, 1989

Not being able to tell if you're being used is a horrible feeling. I take such chances in my life when I begin to fall for a male because I am not quite sure what he may want from me. Does he want my loving care or does he only want to have sexual intercourse? Does he lead me on, pretending to care while laughing hysterically behind my back about how naïve I am?

Welcome to the real world, Tyra! Relationships are nothing but growing experiences. I just hope to grow until I fully understand how to be a champion at the game.

♡T

when two become ONE

That journal entry was from a long, long time ago. And I can now say that I have finally become a champion at the game…almost. Listen, I'll tell you right up-front that I ain't no virgin. I've had sex. It feels good. But it does not feel good enough to risk getting some STD or to risk my life with the possibility of getting AIDS. And let's not forget about pregnancy. Eighteen minutes of pleasure is not worth eighteen years of pain. Don't get me wrong. Having a child is definitely a beautiful experience, but it's really special when the child comes at the right time in your life.

I really think that it's best just to hold out and wait, because sex isn't going anywhere. But there are people out there who are gonna do it anyway, some earlier than you might think. In our discussion group, the ages at which women lost their virginity ranged from thirteen to eighteen. The ages of the guys they were with ranged from sixteen to thirty-four! But no matter when it happened, everyone agreed that it wasn't quite what they'd expected. The decision to be with someone in an intimate way shouldn't be made hastily or under pressure. A few words of advice from the girls:

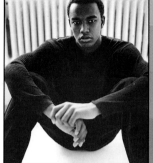

Cheryl: *Give a relationship at least eight months before having sex.*

Monica: *Don't settle for what's kind of good. Be picky. Don't worry about if they like you. Think, "Do I like him?"*

Erica: *Always think about reality. Trust vibes. If you feel your mind is saying no, no, no, listen to it.*

Fannie: *Wait and be emotionally stable. And if you really want to have sex, then just be safe.*

TOUCH, But **Don't** LOOK

We girls obsess so much about our bodies, thinking that all guys want are centerfolds. Not true—those women, as well as my modeling coworkers, are just intangible fantasies. The guys want you. If they didn't, they wouldn't be with you. Even if you've known someone for a long time, it can be kind of unsettling to have him or her see you undressed, and it can create some insecurities:

Erica: *My biggest fears about sex have to do with my body. I gain and lose weight so much that I have stretch marks on my behind.*

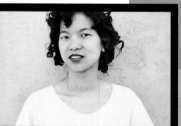

Diane: *I think the reason I'm still a virgin is because I'm chubby and my stomach is big. And I have a big chest and a big behind and I feel like guys are gonna go "Ughhhh!"*

Tyra: *What you just described, that all sounds like what guys like.*

Cheryl: *I know what she means though. I feel that way about my breasts. I don't see why all these girls are getting breast implants. If I had money, I'd have mine cut off. I think I'm a thirty-four DD.*

Tyra: *Well, I have my own insecurities. A lot of society sees me as being perfect. And if I'm with somebody for the first time and they see that I have stretch marks on my butt, and cellulite, and that my waist is not as small as it seems on the* Sports Illustrated *covers, I feel like I don't measure up to their expectations.*

Cheryl: *You* have *those insecurities?*

Tyra: *Heck, yeah! Like, if I'm with a new guy and we're hanging out and he squeezes my waist, I wonder if he's thinking, "Gosh, the pictures don't have this extra piece of flesh in there."*

Cheryl: *Just do it in the dark.*

The idea of having sex with someone you love is that you shouldn't have to worry about things like this. Your partner is supposed to accept you for you, and that means loving the total package. If they start talking about what they don't like and making you feel uncomfortable, then they probably don't deserve to be with you. You probably think you're the only one with the insecurities. But he's probably just as nervous as you are. He may feel that he's too skinny or not "big" enough. So RELAX.

Condom Mania

If you're gonna do it, just take a little time to think about your health and your future. I don't think it's the coolest idea to depend on a guy for protection. If you feel that you're ready to have sex, then you've got to prepare yourself for everything. Part of this preparation involves buying some condoms, or rubbers or jimmy hats or whatever you call them in your hometown. It doesn't matter what you call 'em. Just get 'em and use 'em. Sure there are other options—everything from birth control pills, diaphragms, and cervical caps to Norplant and Depo Provera—and a doctor at any clinic can explain their pros and cons, but condoms for men are the most accessible and the easiest to use. They also provide protection against HIV and other sexually transmitted diseases that the other forms of contraception don't.

Sometimes girls are kind of embarrassed to go out and buy condoms, and many think it's the guy's responsibility. But it's yours too. (I feel funny when I have to buy laxatives, much less something for birth control.) But a little embarrassment just might save your life. So get your butt in that store, pick up those condoms, and look that cashier in the face. And if she looks at you funny, just tell her, "Uh…these are for my friend."

Having them doesn't mean a thing if you don't use them. Some guys will try to say that it ruins the sensation or it does not feel natural. So it's for you to say, "No condom, no sex." It may ruin the moment, but like Fannie said, "You can always get that moment back." But you can't get your life back. I think Olivia, who had been quiet for much of the condom discussion, summed it up best when she said, rather matter-of-factly:

> "If he doesn't have condoms, then you must have condoms. If you both don't have them, then nothing should happen at all."

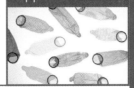

Something for the Ladies

Female condoms are also available over-the-counter, and many women prefer them to the male versions. The difference between the two is that, unlike the male condom, which covers the man's penis entirely, one end of the female condom is inserted into the vagina, and the other end is used to cover the tip of the man's penis during sex. Also, female condoms are made of a stronger material, so they don't tear as easily. Both protect women against sexually transmitted diseases and pregnancy. The only downside: They cost more than the men's. Then again, it might be nice to purchase something made specifically for *our* bodies.

Risky Business

I t is hard to believe that in these times of HIV, AIDS, and other sexually transmitted diseases, there are still people who have unprotected sex. Especially when it's so easy to pick up a pack of condoms. I know a model who went out with this guy who was the biggest woman-chaser. He was obsessed with models, and she well aware of the fact that she was just another six-foot beauty added to his stable. So I asked her, "Are you using condoms?" She said, "No, but if I die of AIDS, just come to my funeral."

Whether you're thinking about sex, or already doing it, you have to think about the risks. On the next few pages I've assembled some facts that cover essentials you should know.

HIV/AIDS HOT SHEET

Where HIV Comes From

The Human Immunodeficiency Virus (HIV) that causes AIDS (Acquired Immune Deficiency Syndrome) is found in the blood, semen, and vaginal secretions of an infected person. It is spread through unprotected sex with an infected person, through sharing needles with an infected person, and, in rare cases, through blood transfusions.

The Number of People Who Have It

According to a Centers for Disease Control report, more than 580,000 AIDS cases were reported in the United States in 1996. Among women diagnosed with AIDS in the United States in 1996, 40 percent acquired it through sexual contact with an HIV-infected or at-risk man.

The Symptoms

HIV can hide out in your body for years without any noticeable symptoms, so you could be spreading the disease and not know it. What is certain with both HIV and AIDS is that the immune system is compromised and finds it difficult to fight off infections. The lower the number of T cells, a type of white blood cell that helps the body fight infection, the more serious the case of HIV is.

The Cure

As of this moment, there is no cure for AIDS. It is not a given, however, that HIV cases will automatically develop into AIDS cases. Medical treatments such as protease inhibitors and AZT or other drug combinations have been known to help, but they are not miracle cures. There are some preventative measures you can take to minimize the possibility of contraction: condoms used with spermicide for vaginal sex; dental dams for oral sex.

Taking the Test

I know, I know. The thought of taking an HIV test is scary. No one wants to hear that they are infected. But think about what's at risk: If you catch the virus early enough, you could start a program of treatment that could prolong your life. By avoiding the unknown, you could spread the infection to your partner or an unborn child. For your own peace of mind, it's better to face the issue head-on.

You can go to a clinic or a private doctor's office to take the test. Make sure you choose a place you can trust and be assured that the results will be completely confidential. They will take a blood sample to determine if you are infected with HIV. It will take some time to get the results back. The other option is to use a company that administers the test by mail; they also guarantee complete confidentiality.

If the results are negative, you may still want to be tested again in six months to be certain, especially if you've been involved in risky behavior. Then if you find that you are free of HIV, count your blessings and resolve to be more careful.

If you find out that you are HIV positive, know that there are health care professionals and support groups that can help you deal with the diagnosis. It will mean making some changes in your life that will be easier to make if you have someone to help you through it. Don't try to go it alone. Times like these are what friends and families are there for.

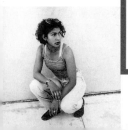

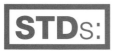

When **S**ex **T**urns **D**angerous

ike AIDS, there is another category of diseases contracted through sex that also deserves attention. In fact, there's a whole list of STDs that can threaten your health. People with multiple sex partners are particularly susceptible. The more you "do it," the more you are at risk. But it's also possible for someone who has only one partner to contract an STD, just as someone with several might. Some people say they are in a committed relationship, so they're not at risk. But let's face it: Sometimes boyfriends cheat, or have old diseases in their systems but have no symptoms. For women, the problem is particularly threatening because many STDs don't have any initial symptoms. That means that a woman could not only spread it to her partner, but in the long run could also suffer severe damage because it wasn't caught in its early stages. And STDs can get pretty serious. They can cause pelvic inflammatory disease, which can lead to infertility.

Knowledge is definitely power.
The chart below gives a rundown of the most common infections:

CHLAMYDIA	Symptoms in Women	Symptoms in Men	Treatment
	Many times, there aren't any	Burning sensation while urinating	Antibiotics that destroy bacteria; have to take all of medication
	More frequent vaginal discharge	Discharge from urethra	
	Pain when urinating		Because partners can transmit back and forth, best if both are treated simultaneously
	Bleeding after sex		
	Pain in lower abdomen		
	Can lead to pelvic inflammatory disease (PID)		

GENITAL HERPES	Symptoms in Women	Symptoms in Men	Treatment
(Herpes simplex II)	Herpes simplex II has painful blisters and open sores in genital area and possibly on cervix	Pain in the testicles	Incurable infection; lesions may go away, but virus remains in the body
		Sores on surface of penis, scrotum, butt, and anus	
	Burning sensation in legs, buttocks, or genital region; tingling in genital area	Discharge from urethra	Treated with antiviral drugs to control the symptoms; ointments to relieve itching of sores
	May feel like you need to urinate all the time; urination may be painful		Should avoid sex during flare-ups

GENITAL WARTS	Symptoms in Women	Symptoms in Men	Treatment
(HPV)	Small bumps in vaginal area or near anus; can grow to look like cauliflower	Small bumps on penis or near anus; can grow to look like cauliflower	Topical drugs, freezing with dry ice, injections of interferon, or, if very large, surgery
			Using a condom helps prevent the spread of warts

GONORRHEA	Symptoms in Women	Symptoms in Men	Treatment
	Many times, there aren't any early on	Thick discharge from penis	Antibiotics that destroy the bacteria
	Infected cervix	Pain or burning while urinating	
	Discharge from the vagina		
	Possible painful itching and burning when urinating		
	Pain in lower abdomen		
	Can lead to pelvic inflammatory disease, ectopic pregnancy, and infertility		

SYPHILLIS	Symptoms in Women	Symptoms in Men	Treatment
	Mild, unnoticeable at first	Open sore on penis	Penicillin
	Open sore around or inside vagina	Swollen lymph nodes in groin area	Can affect heart and central nervous system if not treated, causing heart disease, blindness
	Transient rash (advanced stages)		

If you have any of these symptoms, or believe you are at risk, it's best to get a checkup at a clinic or by your personal physician. Insist that your partner(s) know about the situation so that they may also be tested. It's important to follow the medical treatment to a tee. If you don't, the infection could worsen or could come back. You should refrain from all sexual activity until the doctor says it's okay for you to resume. I've heard advice about talking to partners about their sexual history, which is a good thing, but let's be real: People lie. I feel the safest thing is no sex. Or if you do have sex, USE PROTECTION. I know I probably sound like a broken record, but I can't say it enough.

Please USE PROTECTION. If there weren't so many millions of cases of STDs each year, I wouldn't have to say it at all.

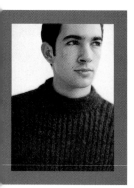

Virginitis

When I talk to women about their virginity, they often say, "I'm saving myself for someone special." I have to admit that hearing this disturbs me. In many ways, this line of thinking makes virginity seem like a gift that should be saved until a man is ready to receive it, instead of a choice a woman should make for herself. I feel that if a woman chooses not to have sex, she should wait until *she* is ready, not until that lucky first guy comes along. Here's what the group had to say about holding on to it, and losing it:

Elaine: *I lost my virginity the night of my boyfriend's prom. What a horrible event that was. But now my views have totally changed. I'm a born-again Christian. I have been celibate for three years. And I don't believe that sex before marriage is the thing that God wants for his young ladies.*

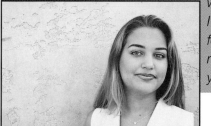

Tyra: *Or young men?*

Elaine: *Oh, yeah, men too.*

Hope: *I was fourteen. It was wonderful. It was everything I imagined it could possibly be. Except the TV was on.*

Deirdre: *I haven't had sex yet because of my mom. I'd get in trouble.*

Tyra: *So you'd tell your mom.*

Deirdre: *Yes.*

Tammy: *My mom said she knew when I'd had sex because she could smell it on me.*

(Everyone laughs.)

Nina: *I was fifteen and I wish it had been with somebody else.*

Tyra: *I think everybody does.*

Janine: *Technically, I still am a virgin.*

Tyra: *What do you mean by "technically"?*

Janine: *I came dangerously close, but then my grandmother's face popped into my head and I stopped. I'm trying to wait until I'm married.*

Jasmine: *I was fifteen. It was weird. I do regret that it was with him. I have a one-and-a-half-year-old daughter because of sex.*

Kim: *I was seventeen. I went to an all-girls high school and that's one of the worst places you can be. And it seemed like everyone around me was doing it, so I did too. But there was no love between my boyfriend and me at the time. So I just got it over with. That was six years ago. When I think about it now, I wish I would have waited because now I have a stronger feeling of what it's like to be a woman and to be in a relationship. And I understand better now about what you give up when you choose to have sex.*

Laura: *I'm still a virgin, but I have a boyfriend. If I ever lost my virginity I'd probably die because my dad would kill me.*

Felicia: *I lost my virginity at sixteen. I've been with my boyfriend for two years and we're still together. I don't regret it…yet.*

None of these women have forgotten their first time. And as most of these girls have said, there really is no need to rush. The decision to have sex is not one to make lightly. If you wait to have sex **until it feels right to you**—not your boyfriend, not your friends—you'll have a better chance of making your first time memorable for all the right reasons.

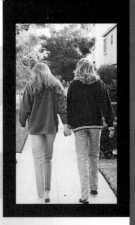

Who Do You LOVE?

"Faggot."
"Dyke."
"Bulldagger."
"Homo."
"Queer."
"Rugmuncher."

Even in this day and age, there are still some segments of society who view homosexuality as a taboo subject, and those who would rather call names than accept the differences of others. Remember what a big deal it was when Ellen DeGeneres "came out of the closet" and declared herself a lesbian? Regardless of the prevalent "don't ask, don't tell" attitudes, I don't think same-sex attraction is something we should just ignore and think will go away.

Of course, the decision to declare a sexual preference is a very personal one. But you shouldn't hold back your feelings just because you are afraid others won't accept you or will call you hurtful names. Whether you believe you were born gay or have made a conscious decision to choose a gay lifestyle is not as important as being comfortable with yourself. If you are gay or lesbian, know that there are support systems in place with people who may have gone through the exact same feelings of alienation or uncertainty you may be feeling, and they are there to listen and to offer advice.

BABY Talk

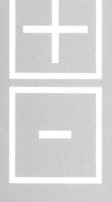

In a perfect world, couples would only have babies when they were financially, emotionally, and mentally prepared to handle it. But as we all know, there are times when unplanned pregnancies occur, and the parties involved are forced to make a decision. The situation is hard enough to deal with when the two people are adults, but when the two are teenagers, the questions become even more complex. So I asked the group, "What would you do if you were pregnant?"

Hope: *I've been through it twice, once when I didn't want it and once when I did. But both times the guys wanted the opposite of what I wanted. So I terminated twice. I think both parties have to agree to have a child.*

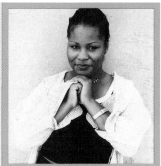

Leanne: *But it's ultimately the woman's decision, simply because you carry the baby for nine months. You have to raise that child. If you give your child up for adoption, you have to live with the fact that you did.*

Hope: *My mom said something to me that will always stick with me. She said, "Hope, you know the baby's father will be there. You know he'll support the baby. You know he loves you. But can you do it on your own?" And I said, "No!"*

Jasmine: *I'm speaking from personal experience. It was my first year of college. My boyfriend and I have been together five years and counting. The first thing I did was call the school nurse, because I knew. I just felt it. It was unprotected sex. She gave me a pregnancy test and, later on, called and told me I was positive. I remember smiling so big because I was happy that the person I cared about so much was a part of me now. Then I hung up the phone and started crying. I never brought up abortion and neither did he. The only person who did bring it up was my mom, who told me that if I didn't get an abortion, the family would DISOWN me. I decided to have the baby anyway. My best friend has had five abortions and her life is freer than mine but my heart is fuller than hers because she looks at my child and cries. When guys see me with my baby, they automatically think that I'm easy and that I'll have sex with them because they see living proof that I've definitely done it before.*

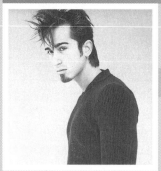

Teresa: *I am pregnant. I just found out last week. I'm four weeks. I'm lucky to have close friends and family to help me with this.*

Tyra: *Are you still involved with the guy?*

Teresa: *Yeah, we're still involved. But I tell him, whether you want to be around or not is up to you. I'm not going to make you feel obligated to stay around because whether you are here or not I'm going on with myself.*

The Pregnancy Test

How to know if you might be pregnant:

1. missed a period
2. breast tenderness or swelling
3. have to pee frequently
4. extreme changes in appetite
5. mood swings
6. nausea or vomiting
7. fatigue

Because these could be symptoms with other causes, it's best to check with a physician. She will conduct a pregnancy test (either a blood or urine sample) and give you a definitive answer. If you decide to buy a kit from the drugstore and do it yourself, be aware that false positives can occur with these tests. A doctor can give you the most reliable information.

Diane: *Now that's a strong woman. I've never been pregnant before. I wouldn't have an abortion if I were pregnant. If women want to have abortions, that's fine, but I wouldn't. Adoption is a good thing. I'm adopted. But I would try to keep my baby. But if I had a baby and couldn't provide for it, I'd give it up.*

Alicia: *I gave my baby up for adoption nine months ago.*

Diane: *My mom said if I ever got pregnant, then I'd have to leave the house. That was her way of trying to scare us from having sex. It didn't work, though. I just know that if I ever get pregnant, I can't go to my mom.*

Susan: *I think it's important for both parents to have a stable income. My boyfriend's on public assistance, so we are waiting until we can support a family on our own.*

Laura: *I'd tell my mom. She's always been there for me.*

Leanne: *I'd go to the guy. I'd want him to know. I would expect support.*

Tyra: *What if you didn't get that support from him?*

Leanne: *(Laughing) I'd call you, Ty.*

The decision to have a baby is not one to make lightly. Too often in our communities, particularly in some segments of my own community, we tend to praise the virtues of having babies without discussing the risks.

Studies show that teenage mothers are more likely to have poor eating habits, or abuse substances such as cigarettes and alcohol, which affect the baby's health, sometimes resulting in low birth weights. Teenage mothers are also more prone to have pregnancies complicated by high blood pressure and anemia. Pregnancy affects other areas of a teenage mother's life, including education and financial welfare. Some mothers have to drop out of school in order to support their children. And without a strong support system, some teenage mothers have the additional stress of raising a child when they haven't entirely matured themselves. For many, the sacrifices are great. You may not be able to finish your education, spend time with your friends, or find a well-paying job that will enable you to support yourself and your child.

I believe that having a family should happen only when you are ready to devote a large part of yourself and your time to someone else, and have enough financial independence to handle the challenge. And there's plenty of time for that. There's no need to rush.

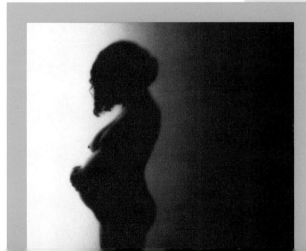

Old **Wives'** Tales

I've heard some of the common myths about having sex, like not getting pregnant if a guy pulls out early or if you have sex standing up. But the whoppers that follow take the cake. None of them are true, of course, but they do show some creative thinking:

Stephanie: *My friends told me to pee really hard after sex and I wouldn't get pregnant.*

Diane: *Somebody told me that if you had sex and he comes inside you, all you have to do is jump up and down and you won't get pregnant.*

Lynn: *I have a girl-friend who drinks hard liquor after sex and swears it keeps her from getting knocked up.*

Erica: *I know someone who stuffed birth control pills up her vagina to avoid getting pregnant.*

F L Y I N G S O L O

When I'm interviewed, I'm often asked what the best and worst parts of my job are. The best is that I have control of my schedule. If I don't feel like working for a week, I don't have to. I just call and tell my agency that I'll be taking a week off. The worst is the loneliness.

I'm constantly on the move, traveling alone from this coast to that continent, from an airport in Argentina to a hotel in St. Barts. And I try to fill the void by reading, watching television, listening to music, and talking on the phone. But it still doesn't completely fill the void the way I want it to. And in the past I've sometimes tried to fill that empty space with having a boyfriend. But when I think about it, whenever I've had a boyfriend, it was rarely my idea. After dating for awhile, I just accepted what they wanted. They'd say, "Tyra, I want you to be my girl." And I'd say, "Okay."

Big mistake. The fear of being alone can make you hook up with people and put up with behavior that you wouldn't accept under brighter circumstances. Ultimately, it doesn't make you feel any better than you did when you were on your own.

The older I get, the more I understand that it's okay to be single. But I'm not going to say it's easy, especially in such a couple-conscious world. Everywhere you turn, there are pressures to be in a relationship. Turn on the TV, and there's a commercial with a couple strolling along the beach hand in hand. Go to the movies, and the screens are filled with romantic happily-ever-after love stories. Tune in to the radio, and there's love song after love song. Go to the bookstore, and there are walls and walls of romance novels. Turn to your buddies, and they're infatuated with some new guy and can't seem to keep their eyes (and hands) off each other.

From birth, women are raised to hope for a Prince Charming to waltz us down the wedding aisle, just like the storybook romances of Snow White and Cinderella we read when we were children. So, to make that fairy tale come true, we make it our mission to find that perfect partner, and when we don't, we feel like failures.

Well, I'm here to tell you that there is life without a man. Fortunately, I have a group of friends I can count on who help me through the times when I'm feeling down about the dating scene. They've taught me that there's a big difference between being alone and being lonely.

Taking on Paris solo

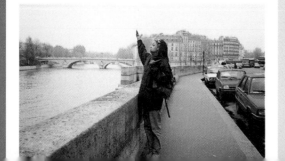

Now when I travel, I concentrate on all the beautiful scenic places I get to visit: the beautiful Seine River in Paris; the gondolas along the canals in Venice; the calm seas of the Caribbean. And I feel fortunate to experience these locales alone. The settings may be romantic, but I don't necessarily need someone there with me to enjoy them.

When it comes to relationships, many of us would do things differently if we had them to do all over again. Here are a few words to the wise from women who have "been there and done that":

"I would wait as long as possible to have sex. I'm twenty-three now and I enjoy sex, but when I was younger, I was just doing it because everyone else was." –**Marie**, 23

"Demand respect. A man will tell you whatever you want to hear and he'll take whatever is offered to him." –**Kim**, 23

"Wait before you have kids, and always use protection." –**Laura**, 14

"I would be realistic. Know that if you have sex with someone, you might not be together two months later." –**Nadine**, 15

"Don't let sex be everything in a relationship because there are so many other fun things to do." –**Karen**, 14

"Your virginity is a precious gift from God that you should give to your husband." –**Felicia**, 18

"You don't want to raise a child while you're raising yourself." –**Jasmine**, 20

"Know who you are. Understand why you are getting into a relationship. Do not look to relationships to fill any void in your life." –**Elaine**, 23

By sitting down with this group of girls and sharing our experiences, I walked away feeling very connected to them. We all came from many different places and backgrounds, but we all shared one thing: the desire to love and be loved. Of course, with that need comes a lot of highs and lows. There will be some heartaches, but I think those times help us to appreciate the good times that much more.

My goal is to find that healthy, love-everlasting relationship that doesn't take over my life, but enhances the life I've already built for myself. I know it's possible, and I know he's out there. But I'm not going to go crazy trying to find him. He'll come around one day.

Until then, I'm going to be thinking about one word: selfishness. Sometimes we don't think of ourselves enough. But it's okay to think of yourself first.

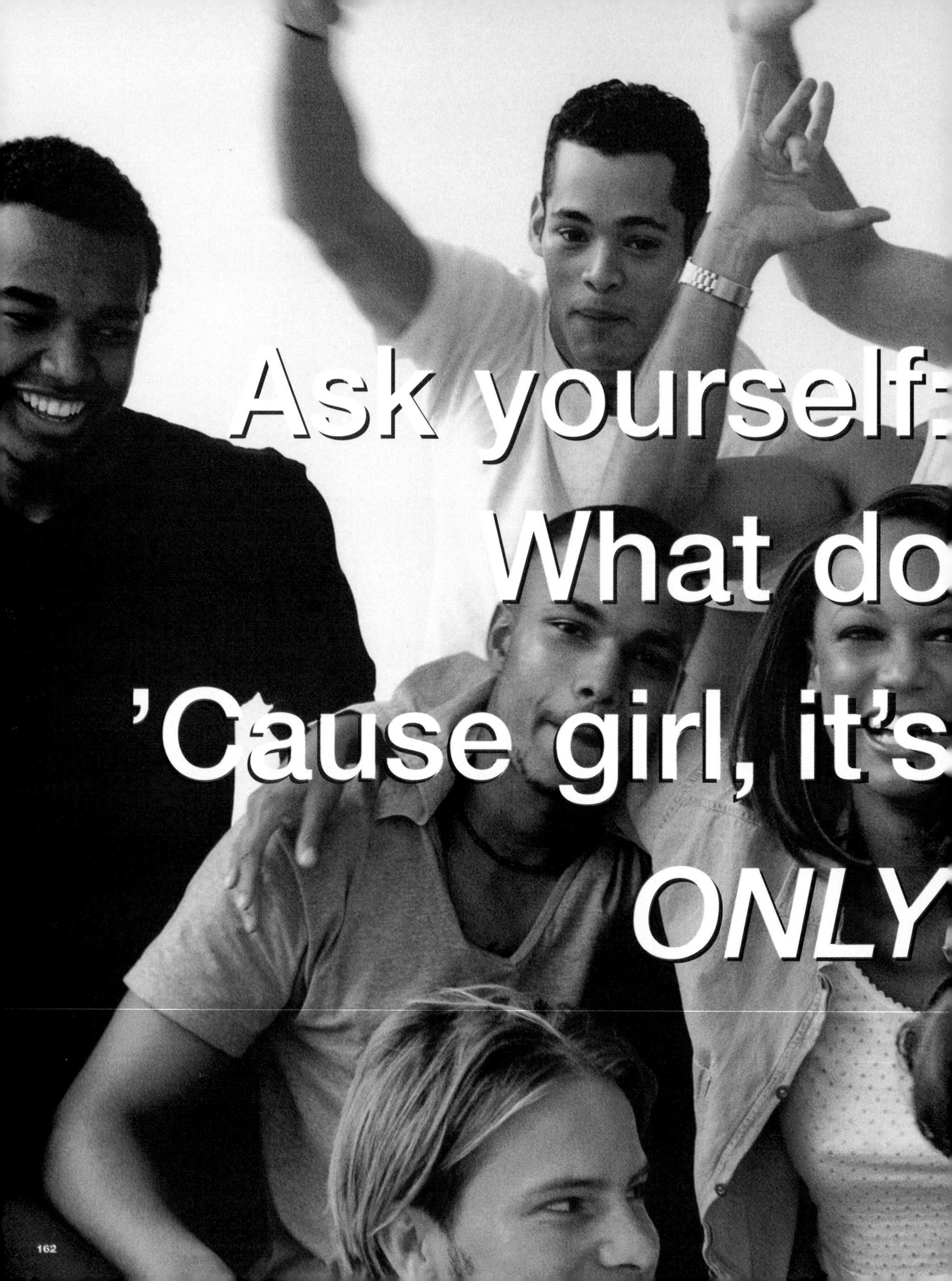

Ask yourself:
What do
'Cause girl, it's
ONLY

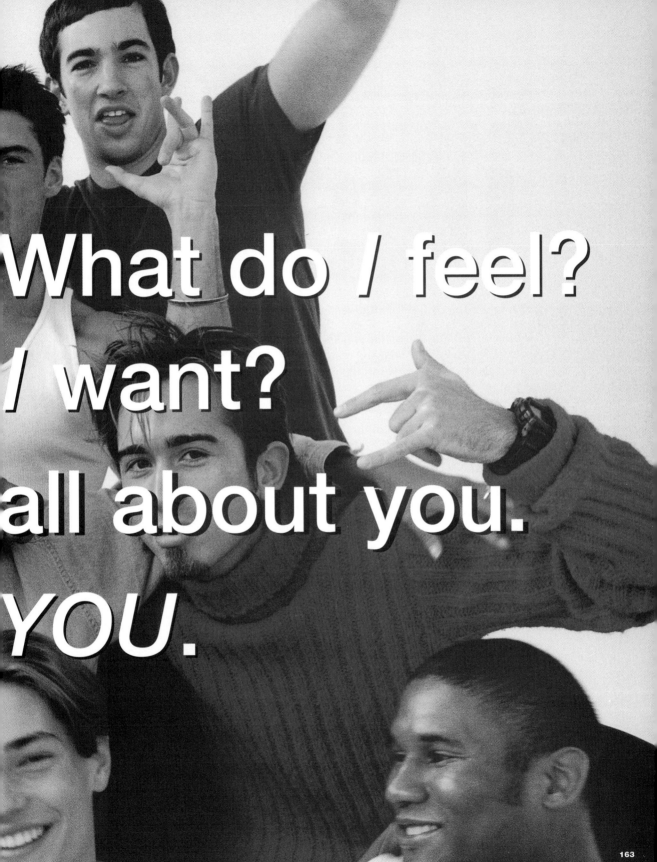

What do / feel?
/ want?
all about you.
YOU.

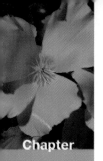

The
INSIDE
Story

I am one lucky woman. I am doing something that I like, and I have been blessed with the kind of career success that dreams are made of.

Some people say that I've gotten where I am today because I had the right *look* at the right time. Others say that I'm just plain lucky— that I was at the right *place* at the right time. I like to think of my success as a combination of things, and most have nothing to do with timing or my physical attributes.

But no matter how many covers I get, how many records I break, how many times I'm labeled a pioneer, it's the letters I receive from young women from all over the world that keep me in touch with reality and what's truly important.

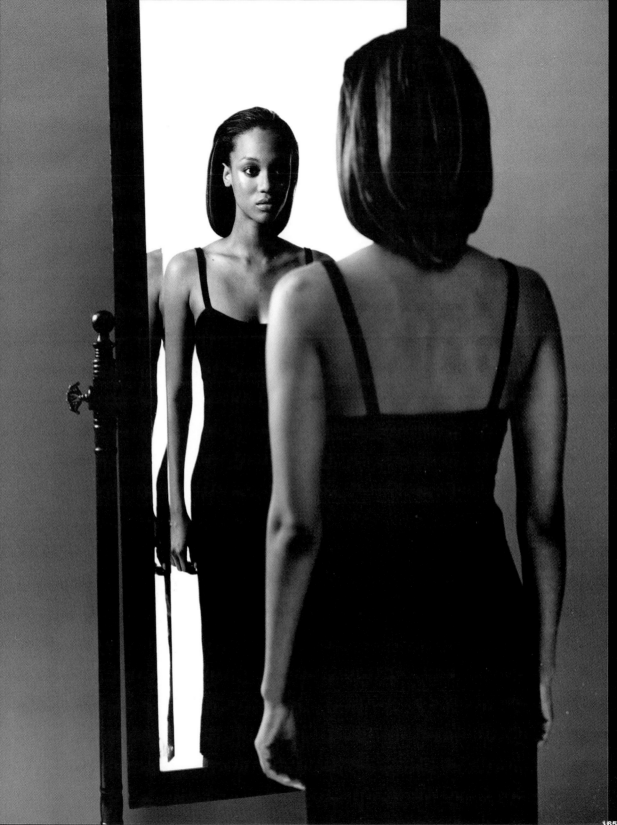

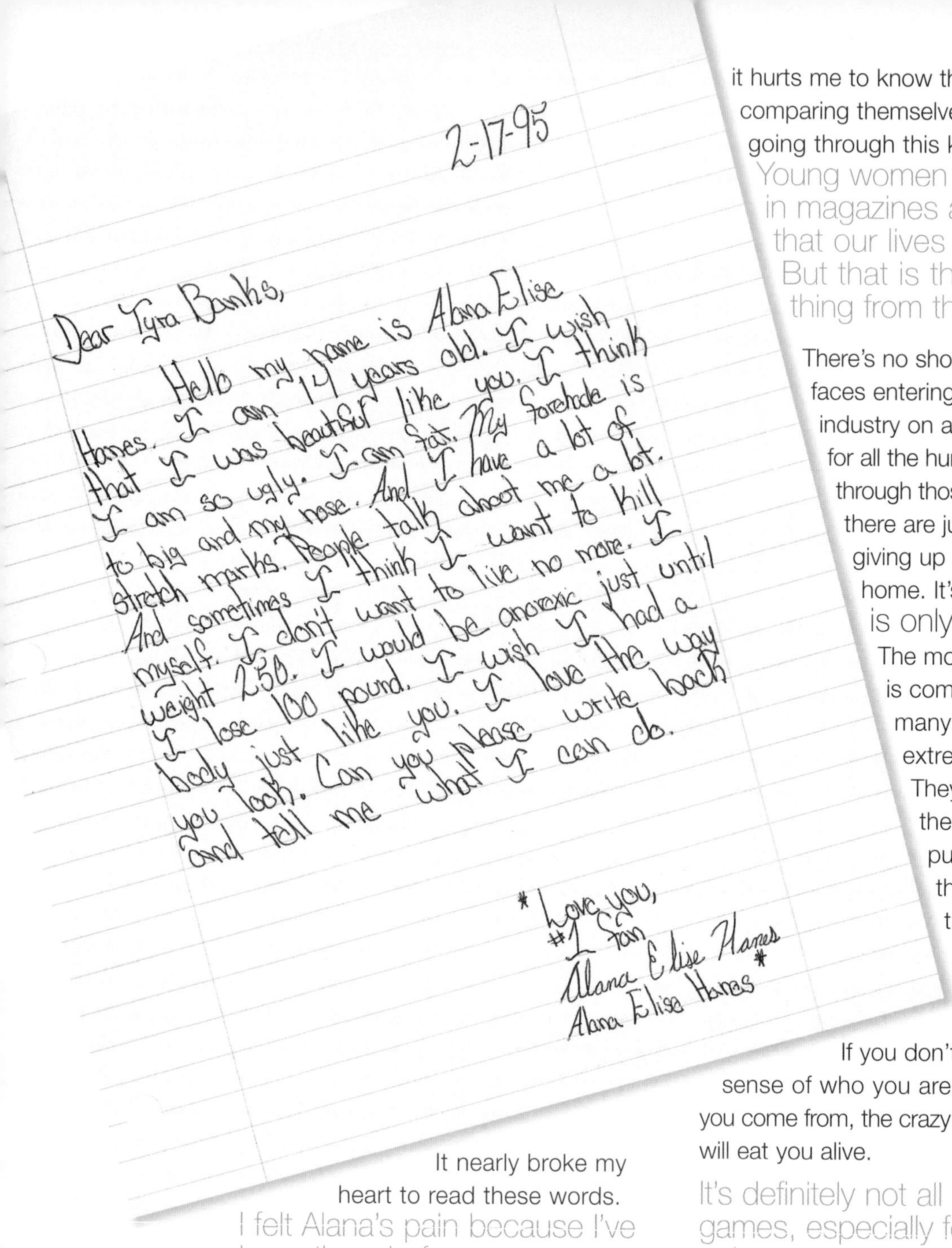

2-17-95

Dear Tyra Banks,

Hello my name is Alana Elise Hanes. I am 14 years old. I wish that I was beautiful like you. I think I am so ugly. I am fat. My forehead is to big and my nose. And I have a lot of stretch marks. People talk about me a lot. And sometimes I think I want to kill myself. I don't want to live no more. I weigh 250. I would be anorexic just until I lose 100 pound. I wish I had a body just like you. I love the way you look. Can you please write back and tell me what I can do.

* Love you,
#1 fan
Alana Elise Hanes *
Alana Elise Hanes

it hurts me to know that women are comparing themselves to me and going through this kind of anguish. Young women see models in magazines and think that our lives are perfect. But that is the farthest thing from the truth.

There's no shortage of beautiful faces entering the modeling industry on a daily basis. But for all the hundreds who walk through those agency doors, there are just as many giving up and returning home. It's true: Beauty is only skin deep. The modeling industry is competitive, and many of the girls are extremely insecure. They worry about their weight, their public images, their looks, and the next hot young model who might take their place. If you don't have a strong sense of who you are and where you come from, the crazy modeling world will eat you alive.

It's definitely not all fun and games, especially for models of color. I learned that the hard way. After a year of my high school friend Khefri trying to convince me that I should try modeling, I finally set out to get signed to an agency. Khefri had already been accepted to a prestigious agency, so I made that one my first stop. The agency

It nearly broke my heart to read these words. I felt Alana's pain because I've been there before, when I struggled with my own insecurities about my super-thin body. The source of my distress did not stem from glamorous fashion models; it stemmed from my community and the value it places on an amply shaped body or physique. Nonetheless, people gave me the once-over and said that I didn't have the look they were interested in at the time. I was disappointed, but decided to just shrug it off and move on to the next place. The second agency said they already had enough girls who looked like me. Then the next one said that my features were too ethnic. The next said they already had a black girl that they were concentrating on and they didn't have the time, energy, or room for another. And the next took my photos to another room, then returned, in less than one minute and said, "Thanks, but no thanks."

Right when I felt like my ego couldn't take another blow, I decided to try "just one more agency." I walked in, handed my photos to the secretary, and waited for what seemed like hours. Finally, one of the agents came to the front office to meet me. She sat down in front of me and said, "Well, Tyra, I see that you have some potential. But I'm only going to have you do runway shows, because I don't feel that the camera likes your face." I can think back on it now and laugh, but at the time I was furious. As upset as the incident made me, I decided to sign with them because at least it was a foot in the door. Besides, I just knew that I would prove them wrong.

In the summer of '91, I did. I vividly remember walking into my modeling agency all happy and excited because I just booked *Seventeen* magazine. But, of course, someone had to break the mood. The receptionist called me over to her and said, "Tyra, honey, you better wipe that cheesy grin off your face. I'll let you know that black models don't have a chance at making it in this industry. So I

suggest you come off that cloud you're floating on and learn how to type. Because next year, you'll probably be applying for my job." Had I listened to her, I probably would have thrown in the towel right then and there. Yes, being black in this business has been tough, but I stayed strong and stuck with it. I don't know where that woman is today, but I'm sure she's eating her words.

I truly believe the secret to my longevity has been not giving in to the word "no" or "can't," as well as my support systems, many of whom I've mentioned in this book. The professional makeup artists, hairdressers, and stylists I've worked with have helped me to keep the outside persona in good condition. But there's an entirely different team who encourage me in my personal life. I'm very fortunate to have such amazing family and friends who see

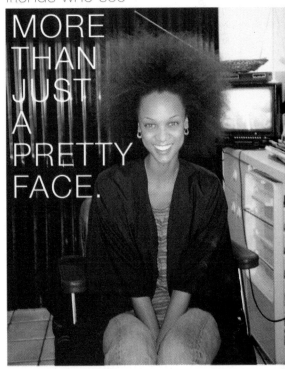

MORE THAN JUST A PRETTY FACE.

A lot of models become insecure because they feel that no one really appreciates their inner beauty. I've made sure that I've surrounded myself with people who help me to keep things in perspective. They remind me that all of the glamorous makeup, outrageous hairdos, fancy outfits, and rigorous sit-ups—the things we've talked about throughout this book—are just a means to an end: feeling good about yourself. That's why I decided I should end this book by talking about a side people seldom see of me: the inside.

Yes, I'll admit, we are judged by how we look; it's a part of human nature. But that's only half of it. Without the inner beauty that comes from a strong sense of self, all we've got is a nicely wrapped package with nothing filling it.

A Family Affair

as crazy as they can be sometimes, I know I can always count on my family. Good or bad, right or wrong, they've been there for me through thick and thin. My parents, brother, grandparents, aunts, cousins, and other relatives have been strong, positive influences in my life, and have helped support and establish me in my career. It's amazing how the love of others can shape your sense of self-worth. A vote of confidence from the home team means more to me than anything an outsider has to say, because I know they have my best interests at heart.

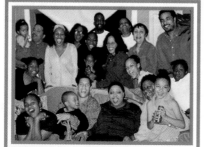
Gumbo party, 1997

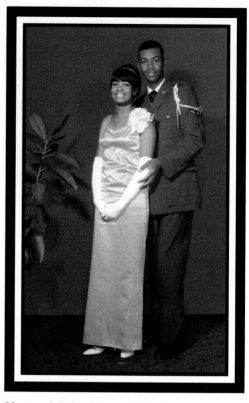
Mom and dad at her senior prom, 1966

My parents married in 1972 and divorced in 1979. I was six years old when they split up. To be quite honest, I was too young to be hurt, scared, or upset in any way. As far as I could see, I had it made. I stayed with Mommy on the weekdays and with Daddy on the weekends. I had two birthday parties, two Christmases. Double the presents, double the love.

It bothers me when I hear analysts try to lump all children of divorce in one group and say that we're so much more likely to be troubled. That wasn't true in my case. I admit I did fantasize sometimes about my parents getting back together. But as I got older, I realized that my parents were better off being apart, and that my brother and I were happier because we weren't stuck in a house full of tension and anger.

I know not everyone can say that. Growing up in a troubled home can be devastating. Sometimes we blame ourselves for the traumatic situation and carry that guilt around with us for years. Sometimes the anger and alienation between the parents can be so intense that children turn to destructive habits such as drinking and drugs to numb the pain.

Whenever I started to wonder if my father still loved me even though he didn't live with us, I would talk to him about it, and he would reassure me that he would always be there for me and that I'd always be Daddy's little girl. It made me feel ten times better. Expressing yourself really works wonders.

It took me a while to learn that lesson with my stepfather. When my mother remarried, it was a difficult adjustment for me. I'll never forget the day she sat me and my brother, Devin, down and told us. I remember feeling like someone had kicked me in the stomach. I felt betrayed. Ma was leaving us. She was going to let this man, who wasn't my father, take her away from my brother and me. How could she?

But then I realized that Ma was in love, and that she wanted our blessing. So instead of whining, sulking, and throwing a tantrum, I put a bright, cheery smile on my face and wished my mom the best of luck, and gave her a big sloppy hug and kiss.

The first few years with my new stepdad weren't easy. He was a strict disciplinarian and allowed no room for slacking off. If those dishes were dirty, I couldn't go to bed until they were not just washed, but shiny, sparkling clean with no water spots. If I was exhausted from a hectic day of final exams and absentmindedly left my shoes and uniform sweater on the living room floor, my stepdad had no problem waking me from my night's slumber to collect my belongings. He took absolutely no crap.

Of course, the strict rules caused some resentment on my part. When Ma was unhappy with me she would complain and lecture, but she'd eventually let me go to bed without doing the dishes, and she wouldn't even think of waking me up in the middle of the night to pick up some clothes I'd left behind. So I started to see my stepdad as a bully, someone who loved to go around barking orders. I ignored all of his positive personality traits, like the fact that whenever I wanted to talk, he would always stop whatever he was doing to listen. Or that he's such a great artist and was willing to share his talents with me, like helping me with my science projects, which were all first-place winners.

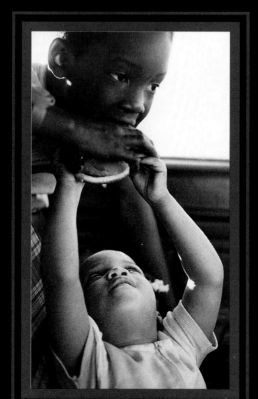

Me and my brother, Devin

The more I took the time to get to know my stepfather, the more I realized that we could relate to each other. I found that when I communicated things I was unhappy about directly to him, it created a bond between us. We became comfortable with each other, so comfortable, in fact, that we stopped running to my mother all the time to settle disputes. To this day, thanks to my stepdad, I can clean a house, cook a meal, and iron clothes better than most twenty-four-year-olds of my generation. I had to allow myself to meet my stepfather halfway. Just that little step took our relationship forward by leaps and bounds.

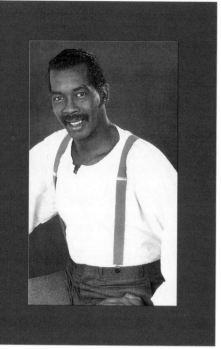

Stepdaddy-o, Cliff

Spending more time alone with my mother also helped me to keep strong ties with her. She understood this and made special time for just me or my brother, which showed us she was not being "taken away" by her new husband.

No family is perfect—mine certainly isn't. The key, of course, is to give and take.

Through open communication I've never had to doubt my parents' LOVE. It's given me a sense of security that I carry with me in everything I do.

Ma&Me

Throughout the book, I've talked about my mother, aka Ma. I've talked about how wonderful our relationship is, how we communicate so openly and honestly with each other, how we're each other's best friend. On the face of it, somebody might think we always get along. WRONG!

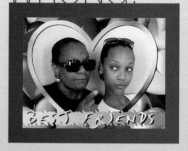

We wouldn't be human if we didn't get on each other's nerves every now and then. Because my mother is also my manager, we frequently have disagreements. We fight, we yell, we scream, and she'll say, "Look! I don't want to work with you anymore! I quit!" And I'll say back, "Fine, I don't care!" And she'll say, "Good, because I'm sick of this!" And then I'll say, "No sicker than I am!" and she'll leave my house all dramatically and I'll slam the door behind her. But before you know it, she calls me on her car phone, snickering, and I'll start chuckling, and then we'll both burst out laughing hysterically because we know how ridiculous we're being and how silly the whole scene must have looked. It's not always this quick a recovery. At times, it can last for days.

So, yeah, mom and I have our battles, but we always make an effort to work them out, and I love her with all of my heart.

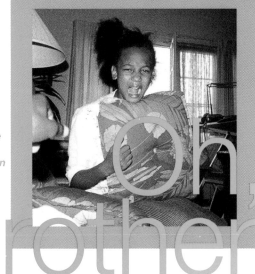

Devin captures the results of his torture on film

Oh, Brother

DEVIN BANKS has put me through more turmoil and stress than I care to remember. I know my brother loves me, but sometimes growing up with him was **sheer torture.** I remember the times he would force me to race my younger cousins, knowing full well that I was awkward, clumsy, and uncoordinated. He took great joy in seeing me trip over my own two feet, laughing as he watched me fall on my face. There were times when I had to literally put up a blockade at mealtimes because he would steal the food from my plate. In response, he would say I looked like an animal covering my plate like that, so I'd release the blockade and of course he'd dig right in. And he always took the meat and potatoes, my favorite parts of the meal, and left me with the stuff I hated— lima beans. I would go to bed with my stomach growling many a night because of this. He was also full of practical jokes. One time I heard a loud crash in the kitchen and ran in to see what had happened. My brother was wincing on the floor and blood was gushing out of his

mouth—or so I thought. I instinctively rushed to the phone and called 911, like my mother had taught us to do. But while I was on the line with the operator, my brother was doubled over with laughter, telling me what an idiot I was as he licked off the "blood" that was actually just ketchup.

No matter how much Devin taunts and teases me, I always know he's got my back. My brother is practically a genius, and he helps me write and do research for my college lectures. He has defended me to the end when anyone has tried to hurt me. If a boyfriend does me wrong, he's the first one to want to kick the guy's butt.

Friends and boyfriends will come and go, but those blood (or ketchup) ties are for life. If you've got a brother or sister in your family, you should be thankful for their presence—even if they can be a serious

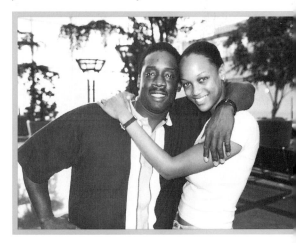

pain sometimes. Next to parents, they can be our biggest fans, and our ultimate buddies. My brother and I have been through it all. We've shared our low points and our successes. I can't even imagine what my life would be like without having him around.

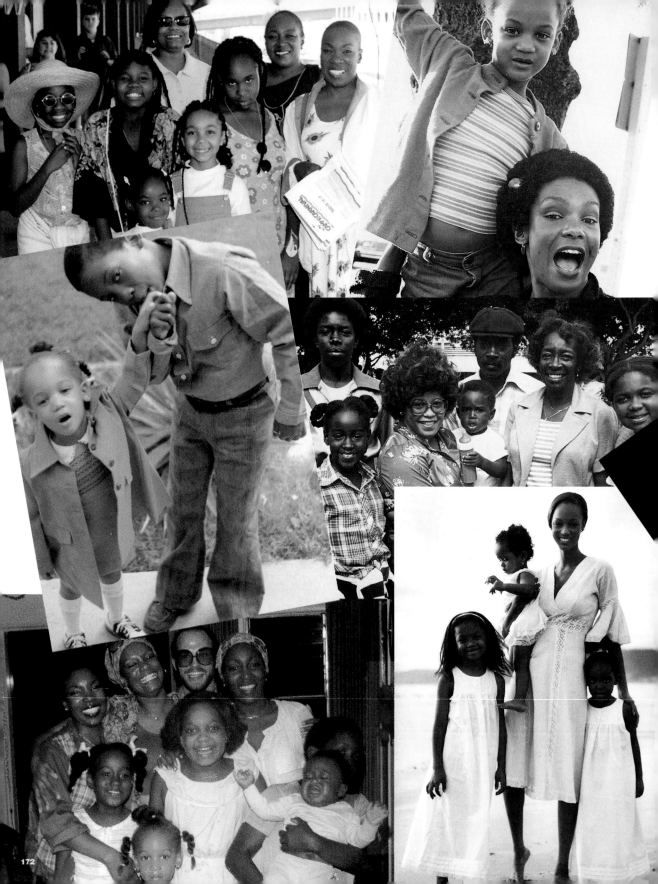

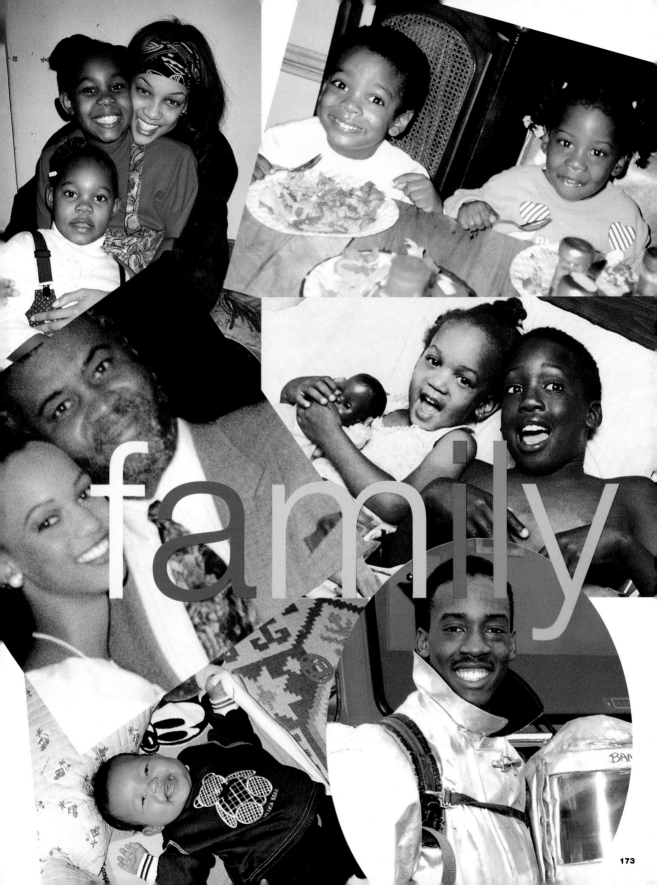

family

DADDY'S LITTLE GIRL

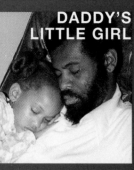

I was spoiled rotten as a little girl. If things weren't going my way, all I'd have to do was cry a couple of crocodile tears and whatever wish I had was instantly granted.

But it wasn't Ma running behind me in a panic to keep me constantly pleased. It was Daddy. I was his little baby. In his eyes, Buster could do no wrong. We spent a lot of time together. Whatever I wanted to do, he supported it, no matter what the cost. I even remember my dad getting peeved when I looked at price tags. Nothing was too expensive for his baby. And I hung on his every word. That is, until I reached adolescence.

Daddy couldn't seem to grasp why I didn't want to hold his hand in public anymore. He was startled when I started to "talk back" and challenge things. (And the thought of me commingling with the opposite sex left him tongue-tied. On one occasion, he refused to shake hands with a guy I was dating.) Yet, all the time he was encouraging me to be the best and to stand on my own two feet, I sure was listening. I was ready to spread my wings. But he wasn't all that ready to see me go.

Now that I'm twenty-four, I'm still not sure what my father really sees when he looks at me. Does he see a mature, grown woman or does he only see his lil' baby still, just stretched out to five feet ten inches with a couple more curves? Well, Daddy, I'm not a baby anymore. I'm a grown woman with a job, responsibilities. And yes, I've had a boyfriend, or two, or three… But no matter what I say, I know you'll always think of me as your little girl, so I guess I'm just wasting my breath.

Don't Let 'Em Get You Down

When I think about the things some of my friends have been through with their families, I am so thankful for what I have. Not everyone is surrounded by such supportive relatives. I had a friend in high school named Kelly who had the worst self-image. She constantly ragged on herself by saying things like, "Oh, God, I'm so stupid. I'm an idiot, just plain ignorant" or "I'm horrible at everything and good at absolutely nothing." To all outward appearances, she looked perfectly fine, so I couldn't understand where this self-loathing was coming from.

One day I found Kelly crouched underneath the cafeteria stairs, crying. I walked over to her and tried to comfort her, but she stopped me dead in my tracks, yelling, "Get away from me, Tyra!" When I asked her what was wrong, she just shouted, "Don't pretend to care about me. There's no reason for me even to exist!"

At first I was startled, but then I realized that she was obviously dealing with a lot of pain. And I just had to get to the root of it. I didn't have a clue as to how to handle the situation, but I did know that Kelly needed help, so I went with my first gut feeling and crouched down underneath the staircase with her. I took her into my arms and just held on tight. By the time she was able to compose herself enough to talk to me, I discovered the source of her pain: her father.

Kelly's father thought he was a good dad. He was a good provider for the family and was present every day. In his opinion, that was the definition of a good father. What he didn't realize was that he was destroying his daughter. He constantly told her that her 3.8 grade-point average wasn't high enough, that she couldn't think her way out of a paper bag. He called her "dumbo" or "airhead" in public, and often said he wished she had been born a boy instead of a "stupid girl." Kelly also told me that when he wasn't making these degrading remarks, he totally ignored her, as if she didn't exist. Kelly's mother was a very passive woman who knew what was happening to her daughter, but felt powerless to do anything to stop her husband from this mental abuse.

I'll never forget how helpless I felt after Kelly shared all of this with me. She begged me not to tell anyone, and I kept my promise. I tried to let her know that I cared, and that there were many other people who could help her if she let them.

Unfortunately, Kelly and her family moved out of the state that summer, and I never heard from her again. I've often wondered if she was so brainwashed by her father that she was blind to the fact that there were others she could have turned to— a teacher, a minister, another relative. It was obvious that she and her mother had very poor lines of communication. They kept silent about the mistreatment and never really discussed their emotions.

That was the biggest mistake they could have made. When I think back to my relationship with my stepfather, I realize that if we hadn't talked about it, our situation could have escalated into something very negative and painful.

Opening up to me was a good start, and I wish she hadn't moved because I know I could have gotten her to share her problems with someone who could really have helped her. I just wish I had recognized the signs that something was wrong earlier on. Sometimes we get so caught up in our own lives that we don't see what other people are going through.

I can't begin to imagine what it was like to live in Kelly's house. But I could see what it did to her self-confidence. Ever since that Kelly incident, I have made it a point to be more aware and to reassure anyone who reaches out to me for support that I will be there for them. And if I can't help, I'll sure find someone who can. I'm supportive, but I'm no superwoman.

Friend OR FOE?

My aunt Sharon suffered from low self-esteem as a teenager, which is so difficult for me to believe when I see the confident and headstrong woman she is today. She told me it all started with a so-called "friend" who really had a negative effect on her and totally crushed her self-esteem.

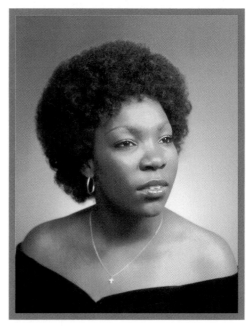

Aunt Sharon's senior yearbook photo

The girl's name was Jennifer. She was tall and shapely, with waist-length wavy hair and flawless skin. Aunt Sharon says Jennifer was the most popular girl on campus, making all the men swoon as she strutted past. Aunt Sharon was new to the school and feeling a bit nervous. She was struggling with a major attack of acne and wore the exact same hairdo every day: a fuzzy ponytail with tightly curled bangs. And her clothes were conservative—a Peter Pan collar, long, pleated skirt, and oxfords—the kind of clothes you can hide behind. One day she was eating lunch (alone as usual) when Jennifer strolled up to her table, seated herself in front of her, and said, "You know, I've been watching you and you've got some really funny-looking teeth. They remind me of a shark's teeth. By the way, I'm Jennifer, and I think I'll call you Sharky. Wanna play volleyball?" Even though she was insulted, my aunt was in awe because the campus beauty had requested her company. She was hurt by the comment and nickname, but no one crossed Jennifer, so she didn't say a word. She just bit her lip, ignored her hurt feelings, and reveled in being the "chosen one" to be the new best friend of Miss Popularity.

Jennifer and Sharon became inseparable for the next four years. But it wasn't a healthy friendship. Over the years, Jennifer continued to proudly attract the male species while my aunt tagged along as her trusty "invisible" sidekick. But Aunt Sharon was changing—she gave up the ponytail for a curly afro. She studied magazines and copied Twiggy's makeup style, false eyelashes and all. She even went on a shopping spree and bought a new outfit for the school dance: an orange miniskirt, white shirt, and white patent leather go-go boots. When Jennifer and her boyfriend picked up my aunt and she hopped into the car with her new look, Jennifer's boyfriend said, "You look so nice. I can't believe it's really you!" Jennifer was so shocked and jealous that she ordered him to rate their beauty and outfits on a scale from one to ten. He sheepishly answered, "Why, baby, you couldn't be anything but a ten." Aunt Sharon says she will never forget that smug, defiant

look on Jennifer's face as she glanced over her shoulder and they drove off into the night.

That was the evening Aunt Sharon decided to sever her relationship with Jennifer. For too many years, she had been ridiculed, hurt, and humiliated by this girl. She wondered why she had been her friend for so long. After ending this unhealthy "friendship," the difference in her attitude and how she saw herself was unbelievable. She was feeling 100 percent better, and all because she'd eliminated this negative person from her life.

I've come across a few Jennifers in my lifetime, personally and professionally. And I have learned that being strong individuals still doesn't save us from coming into contact with negative people and negative energy. There will always be those who attempt to tear us down for reasons that have nothing to do with us. Their mission in life seems to make themselves feel good by bringing us down.

Aunt Sharon did the right thing, even if it did take her a while to recognize the real situation. With every insult, she was allowing her "friend" to chip away at her self-esteem. No amount of popularity is worth what she suffered. All the time you're in pain, that person is enjoying it. As I've gotten older, my definition of a friend has changed, and someone who enjoys my misery is not on the list.

POPULAR POSSE

When I was in the sixth grade I used to hang with a group of girls who I thought were the coolest in my class. As a matter of fact, because I told everyone what to do, I was the leader of the pack.

There was one girl in our class who wasn't a part of our clique. Her name was Sally, and we all thought she was really weird. Even though everyone wore school uniforms, we all thought she *still* dressed funny. All of our skirts were hemmed to the knee, but Sally's skirt came all the way to her ankles. She walked around the playground smiling to herself all the time, and she had no friends at all. She did everything by herself. She ate lunch by herself and even played handball by herself. We thought she was crazy so we always made fun of her, and when we weren't doing that we just ignored her.

My so called super-cool clique had this strange ritual in which every couple of months we'd decide which girl in our group to kick out, for no particular reason at all. And whenever one of the girls was kicked out, she'd immediately become Sally's best friend.

As soon as we allowed that girl back into our group, she'd drop Sally flat. And Sally never questioned it.

Everything was fine until one day the clique came up to me and said, "Tyra, we're tired of you always telling us what to do, so you know what…" I knew what was coming next. And I guess I don't have to tell you who I turned to. As she had done with everyone else, Sally welcomed me with open arms.

Sally and I became the best of friends. I learned a lot about her during the time we spent together, including why she wore her skirts so long (it was a religious requirement). Just as we were becoming really chummy, the so called cool clique came back into the picture and said, "Tyra, we think you've suffered long enough, so you can be our friend again." I'm not proud to say it, but I left Sally behind and went back to the popular pack.

But it was different being with them this time around. I began to see the group for who they really were. They acted like they were so much better than everybody else. I couldn't believe that I was part, let alone the leader, of that. I was so caught up in the pressure to be popular that I couldn't bring myself to leave the group.

Even after the way I abandoned her, when I'd see Sally in the halls at school, she always smiled. I now realize that she was wise beyond her years and understood that I was too weak to break away from the pack and stand on my own…like her.

Thankfully, Sally's kind of self-confidence came to me with time and maturity. I don't belong to cliques anymore, although there are plenty of them in the modeling industry. I used to feel that I had to hang around all of them to be cool and successful, but I soon realized I didn't have to be in a clique to be considered a success. I decided to stay away from the pack and establish my own unique identity. I think I'm a much stronger and more independent woman for doing that.

Thanks, Sally.

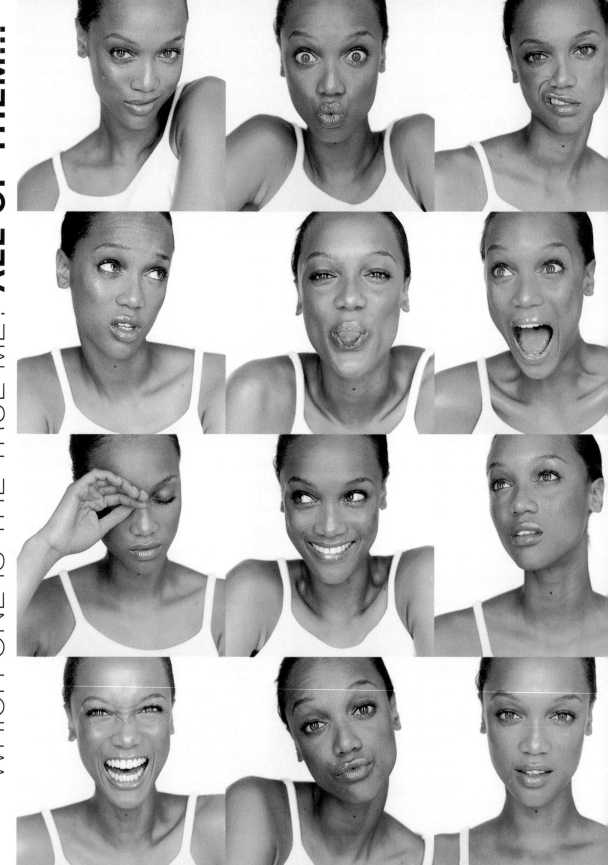

WHICH ONE IS THE TRUE ME? **ALL OF THEM!!!**

4-Give-In

I am a very sensitive person. Because of this, my feelings are constantly being hurt, and I've never been one to "forgive and forget." I'm more of a "never-forgive-and-forget-about-you-forever" kind of girl. Cross me once? I'm gone. Say something that I believe was meant to hurt me? You'll never see me again. I can cut my emotions off with a snap of my fingers.

Some say this is a great trait that I have, that "Tyra don't take no crap!" But the older I get, the more I realize that I'm doing myself more harm than good. When I'm hurt, I tend to retreat and write that person off for good instead of discussing my hurt feelings. I'm always thinking someone is being malicious toward me. I'm beginning to realize that sometimes people are just making small misjudgments or simple mistakes and that this is okay.

They **can't read** my mind.

I have a friend who's been double-crossed, cheated on, and backstabbed more than I probably will ever be in my lifetime. But she is so happy and at peace with herself because she *forgives.* We've all been deeply hurt at one time or another, whether it be a buddy who betrayed us or a boyfriend who cheated. But harboring negative thoughts about people who have turned against us only hurts us.

I saw a movie called *The Ghosts of Mississippi,* directed by Rob Reiner, about the racially motivated murder of Medgar Evers, a civil rights activist. In one of the film's most moving moments, Mrs. Evers, played by Whoopi Goldberg, is having a conversation with her attorney, played by Alec Baldwin, and he asks her why she doesn't harbor any hate against her husband's murderer. She answers, in a calm, composed tone,

"The people you hate either **don't know** or **don't care."**

That line really touched me. It made me realize that no matter how justified we may think our hatred is, we are the ones who ultimately suffer the most. What forgiveness allows us to do is get beyond the hurt and move on. You may not be able to do this right away; it might take some time. Doing it in steps is okay too. Some places to start:

Let it go. If you are hurt, it's okay to store it in your memory, but don't let it consume you.

Make a choice. It is okay to forgive the offender and to choose not to rekindle your relationship with her or him.

Take a chance. You may be fearful of opening yourself up again, but if the person is truly sorry, sometimes they deserve another chance to prove that they value your friendship.

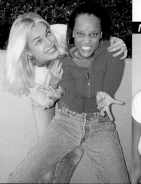
Me and Cassandra

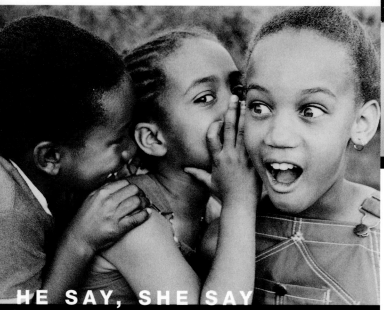

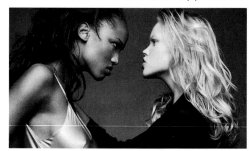
Rebecca and Me

HE SAY, SHE SAY

"Did you hear that Leslie is going with Justin but I heard that she's a ho anyway because Marta said that Sheila saw her with Tony and Robert in the same day and she thinks she is so cute but I hear that all that hair is nothing but a big weave and all those expensive clothes that she wears are all stolen because yesterday I heard P.J. tell July that Jaime saw her in the mall slipping that dress into her bag. Man, I can't stand Leslie!"

Why, oh why do we gossip like this? Get a group of women together and the claws come out. MEOW! (People say that girls are the worst, but I've heard guys talking, and they can be just as catty.) Now I wish I could say that I don't participate in that non-

sense, that I'm way above spouting out the mouth about folks, but I'd be lying. I admit that I've joined in many a time.

One thing I've noticed is that my gossip pattern depends a lot on my mood. If I'm feeling down in the dumps or insecure, I'll be the first to start in dishing somebody. But if I'm feeling confident and at peace with myself, I'll either try to defend the poor victim we're attacking or I'll just leave the room to get away from such negative talk.

Talking about people seems to make us feel better about ourselves. We use finding fault in others as a quick fix to relieve our own insecurities. How many times have you been looking at the television or a magazine and just blurted out that the

glamorous movie star staring back at you is probably a "bitch" or swore up and down that she had a nose job, collagen lip injections, and liposuction from her head down to her toes?

If you take any kind of pleasure, no matter how slight, in criticizing your friends, stop and ask yourself why. Feeling insecure is normal. We all go through bouts of it occasionally.

But, in the long run, talking ill of others only makes you look petty and small. It's better to take the high road. If you are feeling bad, try giving someone else a compliment instead of an insult. The smile you get back won't only make their day–it just might make yours too!

Forever Friends

There's a saying that goes, "To have a friend, you have to be a friend." I have a small core of friends whom I absolutely treasure. Some of them I don't see every day. I don't have to. We could not talk for months, then I'll pick up the phone and we'll start talking like it was just yesterday. These are the people I know I can count on. It feels good to be around them, and I know I can always rely on them. I may even be a godmother to their children one day.

But as close as we are, there are still times when we don't get along. We disagree, and even have in-your-face fights from time to time, and when that happens, it's

perfectly fine to take a break from each other. We may need some time apart to cool down and get some perspective, but we always leave the door open to renewing the friendship. Part of that means opening ourselves up and discussing our feelings. Then when we come back together, the relationship is even stronger.

Telling my friends that I feel hurt isn't easy for me to do. I've always been reluctant to communicate my feelings to people. I used to think it was a sign of weakness. And I always felt that my friends looked to me for strength, so I could never approach them with my problems. But after a while, they looked at me with resentment because they thought my life must be perfect since I never expressed my own insecurities. It alienated them from me.

After watching too many relationships I wanted to hold on to just wither away, I decided that I needed to start giving more in the relationships. I'm not talking about giving advice or material possessions. I'm talking about giving of myself. Knowing how to ask for support is just as important to maintaining a friendship as giving support.

Many of us don't know how. We get angry with others for not giving us what we need, yet we don't tell them what that need is. We must realize that people don't know how to help if we don't know how to ask. It all goes back to what I was saying before about family relationships—the lines of communication have to be open.

Friends and family are both very important. Blood may be thicker than water, but you need water to survive.

The Write stuff

I don't think I would have been able to write this book without the help of my journals. I've kept them since I was seven years old. I used to write in one every single day, but now I pick it up about once a week, usually when something interesting happens in my life. It not only chronicles the changes in my life, I but it helps me to see how much I've grown and how far I've come.

Writing things down has been the best release for me. It frees me from anxieties, tension, and insecurities. There are days when I'll be going through some tough times and I'll just refer back to my journals—and I'll see how I handled a similar problem in the past. I may go back months or even years.

I think keeping a journal, whether you write it in every day or once a week, **is a present everyone should give to themselves.**

It's for those days when you feel like screaming, but you can't; those times when everyone around you is getting on your nerves and you have to let it out; those days when you need to give yourself a little pep talk; those moments when you've accomplished something big and you want to put it down on paper for posterity. And who knows, maybe one day you'll be writing a book and need some firsthand material!

HANDS OFF!

I had a couple of friends who began dating my exes. We all had an understanding not to touch each other's old flames, but they broke that pact. The women who did this to me were two of my closest buddies. Needless to say, we're no longer friends.

The quickest way to ruin a friendship is to date an ex-boyfriend of a friend. If you value what the two of you have, ask yourself if it's worth losing it over a guy who may or may not be in the picture a few months down the line.

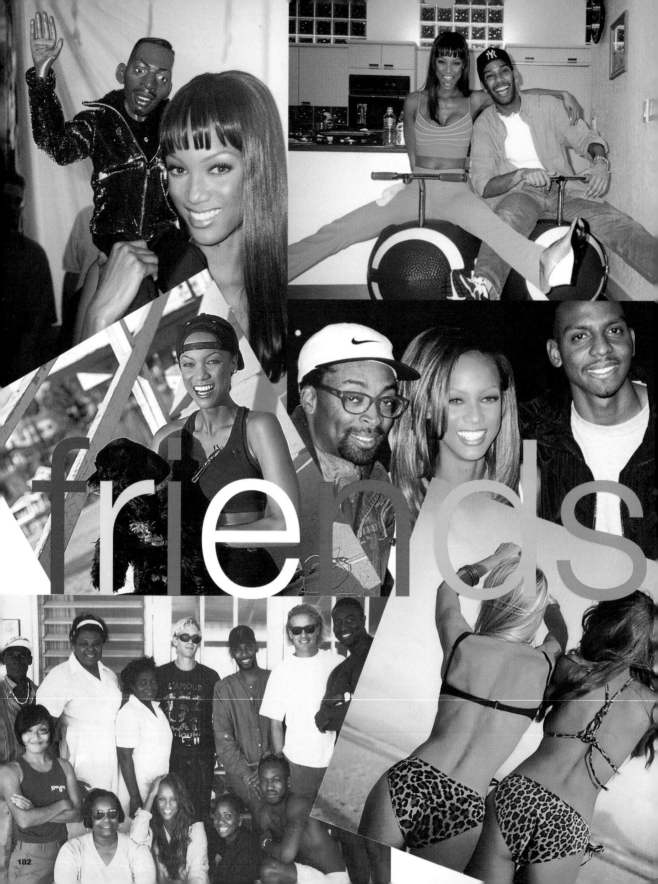

friends

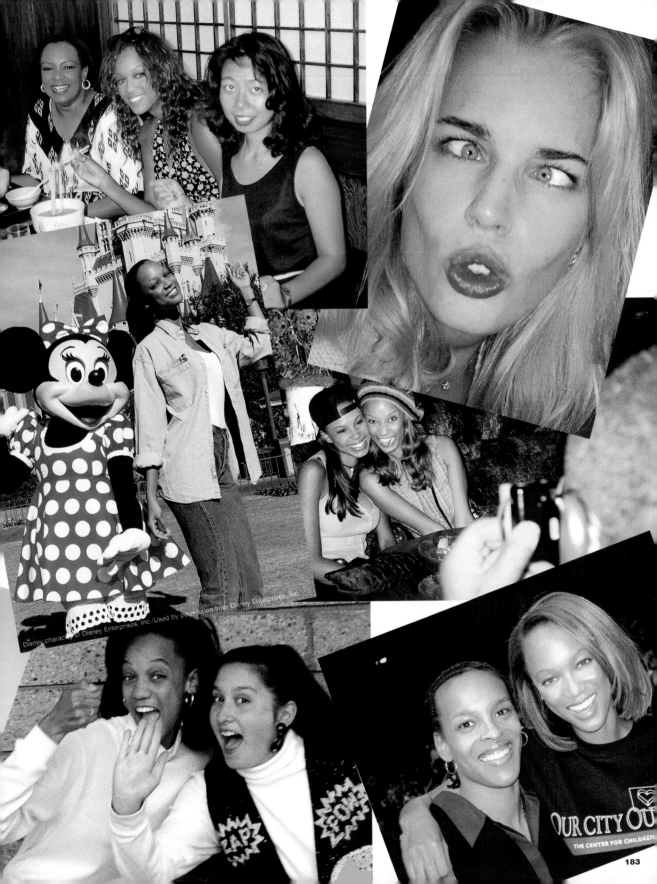

Disney characters © Disney Enterprises, Inc./Used by permission from Disney Enterprises, Inc.

183

Think Happy

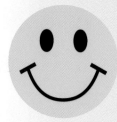

I have days when it seems as though my whole world is about to crumble. I may be on the set of an eighteen-hour commercial shoot in Israel, with a bad case of gastritis, the director is yelling at me because I keep flubbing my lines in Hebrew, and I just got a call from someone telling me that my boyfriend is cheating on me! It's enough to make anyone feel down in the dumps.

But I don't allow myself to go there. What I've learned to do to get through times like these is to visualize being somewhere else. I call it "looking to the other side." While people on the set are scrambling all around me, stressing out, I picture myself alone in my hotel room, far away from the screaming director. The French doors leading to the balcony are wide open, allowing a cool breeze to sweep through the room while I recline on a chaise longue eating a pint of coffee Häagen-Dazs ice cream. With a little gas medication, my stomach cramps are a distant memory. As I lie there, I envision myself being wooed by the most desirable man on earth while my soon to be ex-boyfriend is banished from the planet and sent into exile somewhere on Mars. As I fantasize, the worry lines disappear from my forehead, and my annoyed frown turns into a smile. Suddenly nothing can get to me. Of course, the people around me can't imagine why I have this spaced-out grin on my face. It's my little secret.

Helping Hands

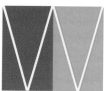henever I'm feeling down and out, the one thing I know that will make me feel good about myself is helping someone else. Many times celebrities just lend their names to a pet project, but I like one-on-one contact. Just seeing a smile on a child's face brightens my day.

My favorite charity is the Center for Children & Families in New York City. I love it so much I've become a spokesperson for them. They work with at-risk youth in all aspects of their lives, from providing housing and food to literacy classes to drug treatment. I truly get so much satisfaction out of spending time with the kids. They're like my surrogate children. We read together and paint together and every Valentine's Day they give me a huge stack of cards—I've wallpapered one wall in my house with them. I spend so much time with the kids that now they are not the least bit impressed by my celebrity. There is no shame in their game. They are so comfortable with me, they even let me know when they think I have on too much makeup on TV. (One kid, Jonathan, compared my new rust-colored makeup to looking like a shiny copper penny.)

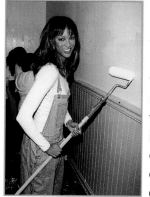

We had a wall-painting party there not too long ago and I was surprised by how many volunteers came in to help us out. That's one of the best parts of being a celebrity, to me, because it encourages others to become involved. I'm happy that I can have that kind of positive influence on people.

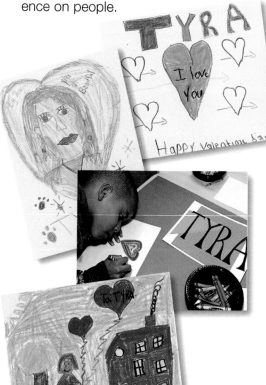

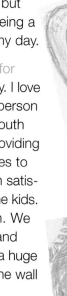

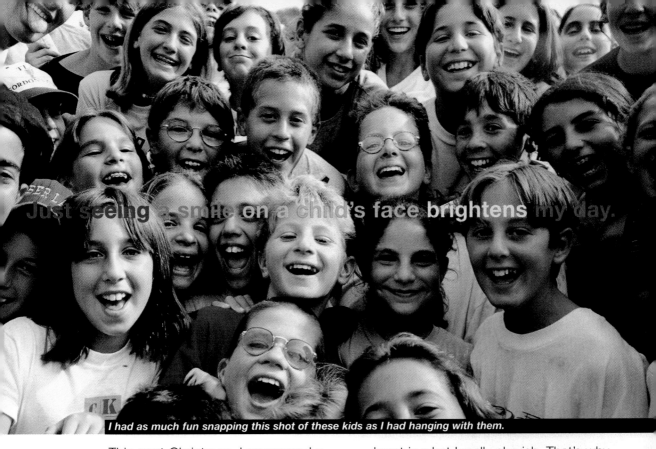

Just seeing a smile on a child's face brightens my day.

I had as much fun snapping this shot of these kids as I had hanging with them.

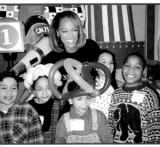

This past Christmas, I sponsored a Kidshare toy drive that was as much fun for me as it was for the kids! I wanted the children from the center, who may have the desire but not the financial means to give someone a gift, to experience the spirit of giving. So we asked corporations and the general public to donate toys, and then we had each child give a gift to another child. I wish I could describe how seeing all those happy, excited faces made me feel, but I don't think words would do it justice.

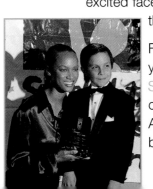

For my work with children, last year I was recognized by the Starlight Children's Foundation of California with its Friendship Award. The award is awesome, but what these kids do for my heart is what I really cherish. That's why I try to do something year-round; during the summer, I visit and make speeches at kids' camps. I'm pen pals right now with a young girl I met through the Make A Wish Foundation. She called me because it was her wish to meet me. I was so flattered that she chose *me* out of all the celebrities she could have met. And when we finally got together, I was even more in awe of her. She has sickle cell anemia, yet she is so upbeat and gung ho about life. Her positive attitude really makes me think twice when I'm complaining about something that's going wrong in my life.

So it really is true what people say: When we volunteer our time and talents to help others, we're the ones who truly benefit.

Dec. 3, 1993

Dear Diary,

I went to visit a man, Theo, a couple of months ago. He was dying. He had AIDS. Theo's mother, Claudia, used to work with my mom at her old job before my mom started managing my career. Theo was a big fan of mine, so his mother thought it would be a good idea for me to give him a surprise visit at their home. I've participated in many AIDS fund-raisers and have taken part in various AIDS awareness projects. And although my mother was a medical photographer for fifteen years, so I saw photos of AIDS patients on a regular basis, I have never visited patients one on one, so the fear of the unknown made me quite nervous.

On the way to Theo's home in Duarte, my mom must have sensed my apprehension, so she took me to a fast-food restaurant to relax me and calm my nerves. When we arrived at Theo's house, we parked and sat in the car for a couple of minutes. Oh, boy, was I scared, but not of the disease. I was just feeling at such a loss for words. What should I talk about? What do I say?

Well...when Theo's mother opened the door, there was a tall, thin, and very frail light-skinned black man sitting on the couch. He looked very weak, but not like he was dying. He was immaculately groomed. His hair was black, bone-straight, shiny, and parted on the side, styled to perfection. The first thing he said when he saw me was, "Ooh, Mama, how did you get Tyra to come over here?" And to my makeup-less face and frizzy, uncombed hair he said, "Ooh, girl, you are so beautiful in person." And boy did that make me smile, because I thought I looked like a monster at that moment. My mom and I sat and talked, laughed and joked with Theo and his mom for almost three hours. I can honestly say that I had fun. Real, genuine fun. It was an evening that I'll always remember.

Theo died today, December 3, 1993, at 5:30 p.m. surrounded by his friends and family, one day before my birthday. I am sad but not shocked because I know that AIDS is usually terminal. But, I just saw him a couple of months ago and I still so vividly recall hanging out and goofing with him on his couch that winter night. I can't believe he is gone.

♡T

Dec. 4, 1993

Dear Diary,

Wow. It's 2:00 a.m. and I can't sleep. When I was younger I would get insomnia because of the excitement of the arrival of my birthday. But I know that I can't sleep for another reason ...Theo.

Right now, I just realized that Theo is truly dead, not coming back, ever. I'm at a loss for words. I don't know what to say. I can't say, "I'll miss you, Theo," because I didn't know him long enough and I can't say, "I love you, Theo," because I only met him once. I don't know what to say because I feel like every word that I think of will sound idiotic...

"I miss you, Theo."
"I love you, Theo."
Even though we spent only three hours together.

♡T

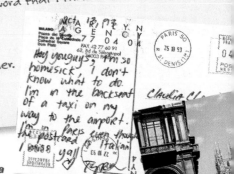

Hey you guys, I'm so homesick, I don't know what to do. I'm in the backseat of a taxi on my way to the airport. I'm in Paris even though the postcard yall...

Claudia Cl...

One of the hardest parts of reaching out to ill people is the risk of becoming too attached. But the joy that comes from it far outweighs the pain. I feel so fortunate to have met Theo, even if it was for only a few hours. **He opened my eyes, not only to AIDS, but to our shared humanity.** He may have thought meeting me was special, but I'm the one who will **ALWAYS** be grateful for meeting him.

GIRLS RULE!

It was during my second year of junior high school, when my parents decided to send me to an all-girls school: Immaculate Heart Middle and High School.

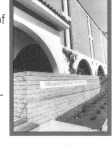

At first, the thought of going to school with only girls felt kind of weird. But over time, it became more comfortable than being around males. We didn't worry about looking "cute" and styling our hair and makeup for hours to impress guys. We concentrated on our schoolwork and campus events and, of course, gossip. It was great to see girls in leadership positions, from student government to team captains. Immaculate Heart Middle and High School is known for developing strong, independent women. Eighty-five percent of its graduates go on to a four-year college; almost one hundred percent go on to some kind of college.

It sure was a lot different from my elementary school days. There was one teacher there in particular who frequently called on the same four boys in class to answer all of her questions. I remember holding my hand up for so long one time that my arm went numb. There was definitely a double standard. If I talked in class, I was called "fast" and was sent to the principal's office, whereas my male counterparts who misbehaved were just "boys being boys."

I don't think it's too far a stretch to think that the other girls in the class and I were being discriminated against because of our gender. Not too long ago I saw a TV special about an in-depth study that proved school-age boys received more attention from their teachers than did girls. It also indicated that boys were encouraged more than girls to excel in math and science.

When women are told that we "can't" do something over and over, or aren't even encouraged to try, we begin to think that we're incapable of doing whatever it is. In reality, all we need is some encouragement. Today I can truly appreciate my parents sending me to Immaculate Heart. I was privileged to be able to attend such a fine school, led by women who were such good role models. Five years ago I established a **Tyra Banks Scholarship** there so that other young women less fortunate than I can have the same opportunity.

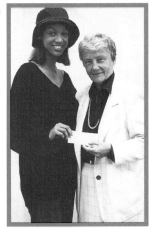

Me and Ruth Anne Murray, principal of Immaculate Heart

Throughout my four years at Immaculate Heart I knew that I was lucky…I played basketball, took wonderful classes, held the position of Junior class president, and met wonderful people. Each of these aspects has made me the person I am. And I love who I am! I know that Immaculate Heart has also instilled that sense of self-love within me.

– **Tina Gardner**
First recipient of the Tyra Banks Scholarship

This scene repeatedly happens to me: I walk into a restaurant and give my name to the maître'd. When a table finally becomes available and I walk up to the desk alone, they rarely fail to say, "Excuse me, Ms. Banks, but we can't seat you until the rest of your party arrives." I always want to yell, "Hey, honey, the party is here. I'm flying solo!"

A lot of people are uncomfortable doing things by themselves. If they can't find someone to tag along, they'll just stay at home. Not me. Dining alone is definitely my thing. But going to the movies by myself is one of the most pleasurable things I do. I get my popcorn, licorice, and large soda. I then make a beeline for my favorite seat, eighth row center.

I'll admit that at one time I was kind of uncomfortable spending time alone. If I dined alone I'd have to bring a book or magazine with me just so I'd have something to do. I thought people were staring at me and feeling sorry for me. Of course, I soon got over that paranoia. Now I challenge myself to do the ultimate solo project: going to an amusement park alone. I haven't done it yet, but just wait and see.

I learned to deal with "solo socializing" at the age of seventeen when I left home for Paris to begin my modeling career. I really didn't know anyone in Paris except my agents and a few models who liked the partying nightlife more than I did. So instead of hanging with them, I took off on my own to discover forms of entertainment that I could thoroughly enjoy without someone to share them with. I visited museums, tried new and unusual foods at restaurants (which was a

departure from my mainstay of fast-food chains), discovered the best ice cream parlor in Paris, lived in the American bookstore, chatted with tourists while people watching at sidewalk cafés. I searched for movies with English subtitles and practiced my French with every shopkeeper in town. I especially loved grocery shopping at unique little places like the quaint butcher shops, vegetable stands, and local bakeries, where every morning

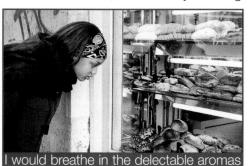

I would breathe in the delectable aromas

wafting from their ovens. I remember the first time my mother came to visit me in Paris. She was shocked and totally impressed with the fact that I had become so independent and had learned so much on my own.

Those early experiences in Paris made me aware of my true inner strengths and helped me to hone my survival skills. I learned so much about myself by spending time with myself. It actually made it much easier to deal with all the solo traveling that is required in my modeling career. I spend a tremendous amount of time alone on airplanes, in hotel rooms, and riding in the backseat of automobiles. It taught me to learn about myself, to ask myself questions like: "Who am I?" "What is my philosophy of life?" "What truly makes me happy?" I've learned a lot about me during those times alone, and I still have a whole lot to discover. Maybe that trip to the amusement park is long OVERDUE.

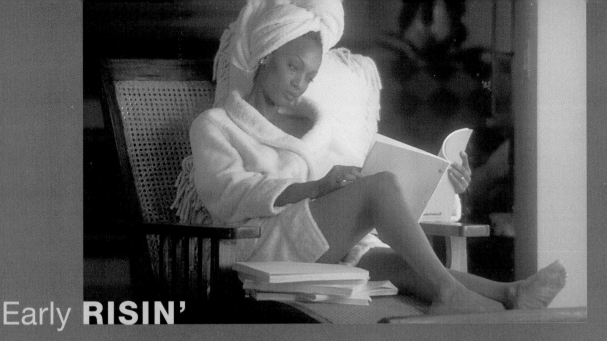

Early RISIN'

I love waking up early. In fact, I rarely sleep past 6:00 a.m., which means I usually get to bed no later than 10:00 p.m. My friends make fun of me for going to bed early, but there's a method to my madness.

I don't necessarily jump right out of bed. Sometimes I just lie in the bed for an hour—no television on, no radio playing. I just stare at the ceiling and let my mind wander. Other times, I get out of the bed, wrap myself in my favorite terry cloth robe, and gaze out the window.

It's so beautiful that I want to share it with someone, but I've learned not to call my friends as soon as I wake up. Not everyone is a morning person. The sound of their phones hanging up in my ear has been a lesson that I should wait until a "decent" hour to call. My best friend doesn't even wait for me to say a word. She just answers the phone without a greeting and says, "Tyra, have mercy, girl!"

They don't know what they're missing: the early-morning sounds of birds singing, the wind rustling the leaves in trees, the neighborhood clinks and clatter as people slowly start their mornings. The quiet serenity of those early-morning hours energizes me. I take time to be thankful for what I have and just for having another day to be with the people I love. It also makes me more productive, because it gives me time to clear away the clutter in my mind. Once that's done, I can focus on the day ahead.

You don't necessarily have to get up at the crack of dawn to take time for yourself. Setting aside a few moments each day to feed your inner self is essential—it better enables us to cope. While you're running around doing things for everyone else, make time to do something for yourself. You can use the time any way you want—to go for a quiet jog, meditate, pray, do needlepoint, or take a nap. It doesn't matter what you do, just do it, because you deserve a little time for yourself—everyone does.

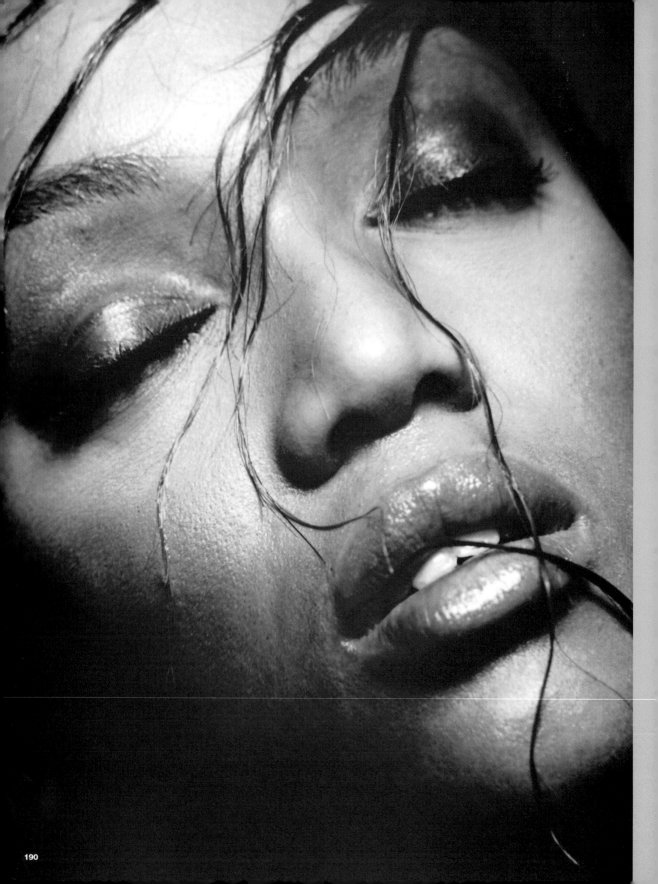

HEAVENLY WICKS AND WAX

When people enter my home, they instantly realize one of my true obsessions: candles. I have candles in every room–short ones, tall ones, skinny ones, colorful ones, scented ones, dripless ones, comical ones. There's nothing like coming home after a long and stressful day and turning off all the electric lights and burning my candles. When that warm, amber light starts to flicker and the soothing aroma begins to fill the room, the memories of my strenuous and tedious day come to a halt. My mind relaxes and I begin to feel at ease. My favorite place to burn them is in the bathroom. I have a glass-enclosed shower and I often light vanilla-scented candles just outside it to put me in a mellow mood. I also love to set them along the edge of the bathtub and let them burn while I soak in a warm bath filled with fruit-scented bath oils. Candlelight is calming. It allows you to reflect, to let your mind wander. But don't wander too far away–leaving candles unattended is dangerous.

I've always had my mom to look up to, but she wasn't my only idol. When I was a little girl, there was a black anchorwoman in Los Angeles named Angela Black, who I wouldn't miss watching on the news. Just by seeing her face each day, knowing that she probably had to beat many odds to make it to this level of her profession was an inspiration to me. She made me believe that if she could be successful and reach her goals, so could I.

There are countless women in the public eye who encourage us to be our best by the fine example they set both in their approach to their work and in the way they live their lives. Here are a few of my favorites:

GLORIA ESTEFAN
Not only is she an incredible vocalist, but she also went through a terrible accident and made a remarkable recovery, all the while staying strong and never losing faith.

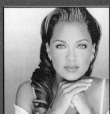

VANESSA WILLIAMS
Full of strength and perseverance, she proved that everyone who doubted her was dead wrong. Success is always the best revenge.

OPRAH WINFREY
Even though she is one of the richest women in the world, she is still one of the "realest," most down-to-earth people you'd ever want to meet. Everyone can relate to her, which is a wonderful quality to have.

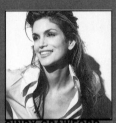

CINDY CRAWFORD
She was the first to make everyone understand that modeling is a business, and for that she is one of the most respected women in the industry.

MAYA ANGELOU
Her writing transcends all races, all boundaries, and touches everyone. No one who reads her powerful words can walk away untouched.

CHELSEA CLINTON
Even though she is the President's daughter, she is definitely her own person. And she does an excellent job staying as normal as possible while her life is being documented everywhere.

BARBRA STREISAND
People tend to put women down who show strength and know what they want, but those are the traits I admire in her.

MARGARET CHO
Her brand of comedy is strictly take-no-prisoners. She's not afraid to say what's on her mind, plus she's just downright funny.

TONI MORRISON
She writes with such strength and beauty that it is easy to see why her work won the Nobel Prize for Literature.

JENNIFER LOPEZ
A very talented actress, she is making her mark in film by choosing compelling roles that give greater exposure to Latin cultures.

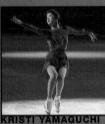

KRISTI YAMAGUCHI
Although ice-skating has lost some of its luster in the past few years, she is one of the few Olympic champions to retain the grace and beauty of the sport.

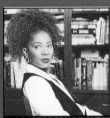

TERRY MCMILLAN
She broadened the audience for black literature and got people who had never opened a book to read.

CHERYL MILLER
Back in the day, my dad took me to a USC basketball game where she was the star athlete. She opened doors for women in basketball. Because she was so tall and thin, she was also a good role model for me as I struggled with my body image. Now she's the coach of the WNBA's Phoenix Mercury.

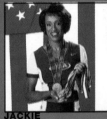

JACKIE JOYNER-KERSEE
She has asthma, yet learned how to work through that to become the best athlete in the world.

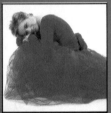

KERRIE STRUG
Her courageous act to help the U.S. Women's Gymnastics Team win the gold medal, even when she was in incredible pain, was one of the most unforgettable moments of the 1996 Summer Olympics.

> **IN EACH OF US THERE IS A QUEEN. SPEAK TO HER AND SHE WILL COME FORTH.**
>
> –"Sisterspeak" column, *Ebony* magazine

LOVIN' ME, ME, LOVIN' YOU

I will be the first to admit that I have my faults. I can be bossy, overbearing, a "know-it-all," I often open my mouth before I think, and I clown around way too much for some people's tastes. But overall, I think positively about myself, because if I don't, no one will. I guess you can say, **I love me some Tyra!** I have not always been as confident about who I am; it has taken a lot of work and is an ongoing project. I'm learning how to move past second-guessing myself, and I'm trying to squash feeling like I'm not good enough, not smart enough, not worth enough. Accomplishing this is something I have to do on my own, with my own confidence and courage. I found that it is truly important to rely on your own instincts to get where you want to be.

Yeah, I may have been really lucky to have a "supermama" show me the way. But now she's stepping back to allow me to become the independent, grown woman she knows I will be one day (I'm not all the way there yet). I get all depressed when my mom starts talking about how she could become very ill or experience some horrible tragedy that would abruptly end her life, and she wouldn't be around for me anymore. And as much as I hate to hear her speak this way, I have to admit to myself that she is absolutely right. I realize that Ma is not always going to be around to come flying to my rescue. So now Ma has begun to prepare me by pushing her baby out of the nest. She's set the stage. She's done her job. I no longer need to play "follow the leader." I'm on my own now. No matter how many times I was told to believe in myself and accept who I am, I had to put forth that effort myself. Because if I didn't believe in me, why should anybody else?

The first movie I ever saw in a theater was *The Wiz.* I was so touched by the song Lena Horne sang to Diana Ross, "Believe in Yourself," that I begged my mama, my daddy, my aunts, uncles, and cousins to take me to see it as many times as I could—I think I finally stopped after the eighth time (but then would later watch it over and over when in came on television). I'm still captivated by the words:

Believe in yourself right from the start

Believe in the magic right there in your heart

Believe all these things, not because I told you to,

If you believe in yourself

Just believe in yourself

As I believe in you

By going through some challenging experiences on my own, I now understand the importance of what I like to call *self-loving.* To me, self-love is the real approval and appreciation of who we are deep down inside. I'm not talking about that "I'm so cute. I'm so fine. I'm all that and a bag of chips" kind of self-love. We are all we've got, so we better get to lovin' not only who we see in that mirror but what we feel about ourselves when we look in that mirror.

Hey, I know I ain't perfect. And it's okay. I'm dealing with so many different issues (so many that I could write a Volume II to this book). And I'll say it again: It's okay, as long as I keep loving myself.

SELF-LOVE has very little to do with how you feel about your outer self. It's about accepting *all* of yourself. You've got to learn to accept the fool in you as well as the part that's got it goin' on.

♥ Tyra

Make a little pampering a part of your daily regimen.

– Chapter 1 **Head-to-Toe Glow**

The key to any makeup routine is to keep it real.

– Chapter 2 **Makeup Skillz**

Hair responds to care, but it also responds to neglect.

– Chapter 3 **Turning Heads**

Make a commitment to eat to live— not live to eat— and stay active.

– Chapter 4 **Body Language**

Follow fashion, but *don't* be a slave to it.

– Chapter 5 **Fashion 411**

If something feels too good to be true, it probably is.

– Chapter 6 **Flying on a Natural High**

Give him some space— and demand your own.

– Chapter 7 **SeX-Rated**

It's all about lovin' not only *who we see* in the mirror but *what we feel* about ourselves when we look in the mirror.

– Chapter 8 **The Inside Story**

Hot Lines

It's always great to turn to family and friends when we need help, but sometimes we may need outside help to cope with some of our problems.

Sometimes we just need a sounding board, someone to listen who is objective and non-judgmental, who will offer advice and support whenever we need it. Below I've listed the names and phone numbers of several national organizations that provide information, encouragement, and support. These hot lines get hundreds upon hundreds of calls each day, so don't be shy about calling them. And remember, your problem is not unusual or weird to them, so there's nothing to be embarrassed about. It could be the best twenty-five cents (or less if it's toll-free) you've ever spent:

TeenAIDS
1-800-440-TEEN

Centers for Disease Control and Prevention National AIDS Hotline
1-800-342-AIDS

National Drug Information Treatment and Referral
1-800-662-HELP

Center for Substance Abuse Prevention
1-800-729-6686

National Council on Alcoholism and Drug Dependence
1-800-475-HOPE

National Breast Cancer Hotline
1-800-221-2141

Reality Female Condom
1-800-635-0844

National Mental Health Association
1-800-969-6642

Planned Parenthood Federation
1-800-230-PLAN

The American Heart Association
1-800-AHA-USA-1

The American Cancer Society
1-800-ACS-2345

The American Lung Association
1-800-LUNG-USA

National Women's Health Organization
1-800-532-5383

National Domestic Violence Hotline
1-800-799-SAFE

Rape, Abuse, and Incest National Network
1-800-656-HOPE

National Center for Overcoming Overeating
1-212-875-0442

National Association of Anorexia Nervosa and Associated Disorders
1-708-831-3438

Gay and Lesbian National Hotline
1-888-THE-GLNH

Fan Mail

I love receiving mail. Wanna write me? Send your letter to:
**Tyra Banks
15030 Ventura Blvd.,
1-710
Sherman Oaks,
CA 91403**

Wardrobe Credits

Tart, Scala, Susan Lazar, Wolford, Randolph Duke for Halston, Michael Kors, Veronica M for Scala, Jennifer Kaufman, The Gap, Alberto Biani, Romeo Gigli, Dolce & Gabano, J.P. Tod, Todd Oldham Jeans, OMO Norma Kamali, Danskin, Fila, Reva Mivasagar, Country Road Australia, Culture + Reality, Dana Kellin, Michael Smicht, Custo, Vivianne Tam, Emporio Armani, Me + Ro, Amle Arte, Ten Thousand Things, Belle Costes, Wouters + Hendrix, Orly Baruch Designs, Michael Morrison

A portion of the proceeds from the sale of this book is being donated to:

THE CENTER FOR CHILDREN + FAMILIES, INC.

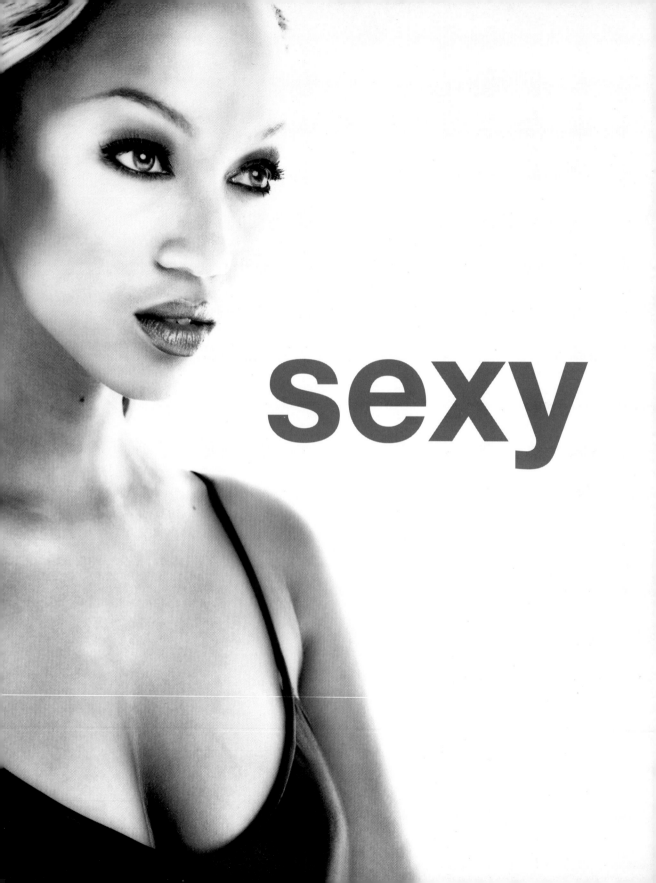

sexy

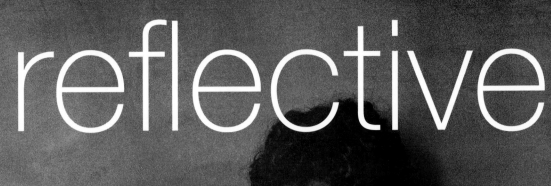

reflective

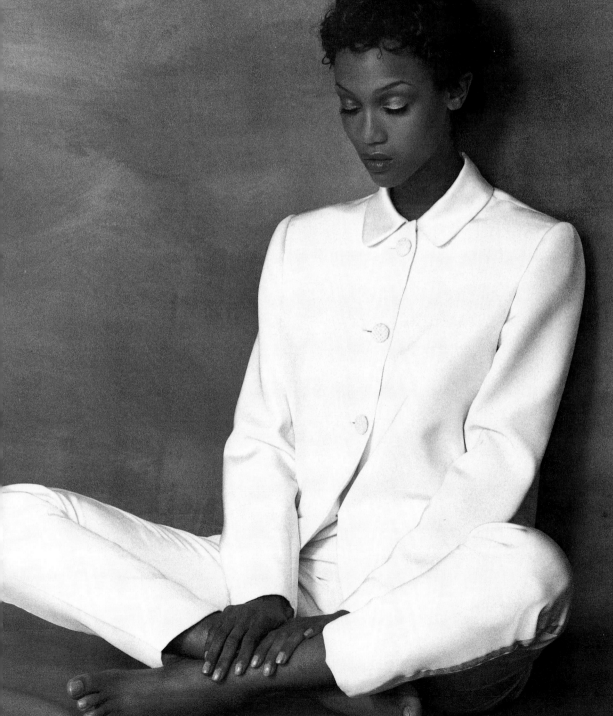

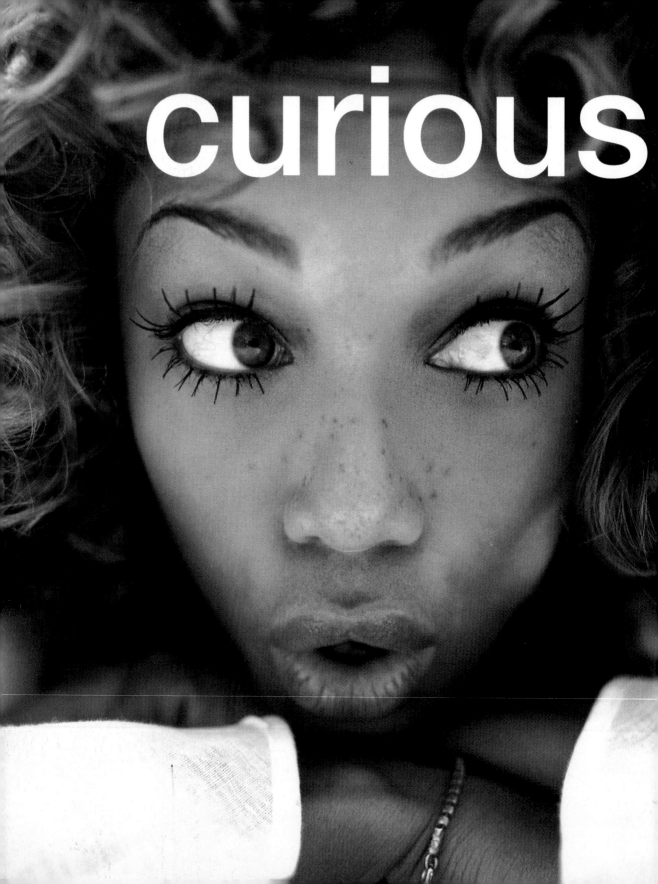

curious

intense

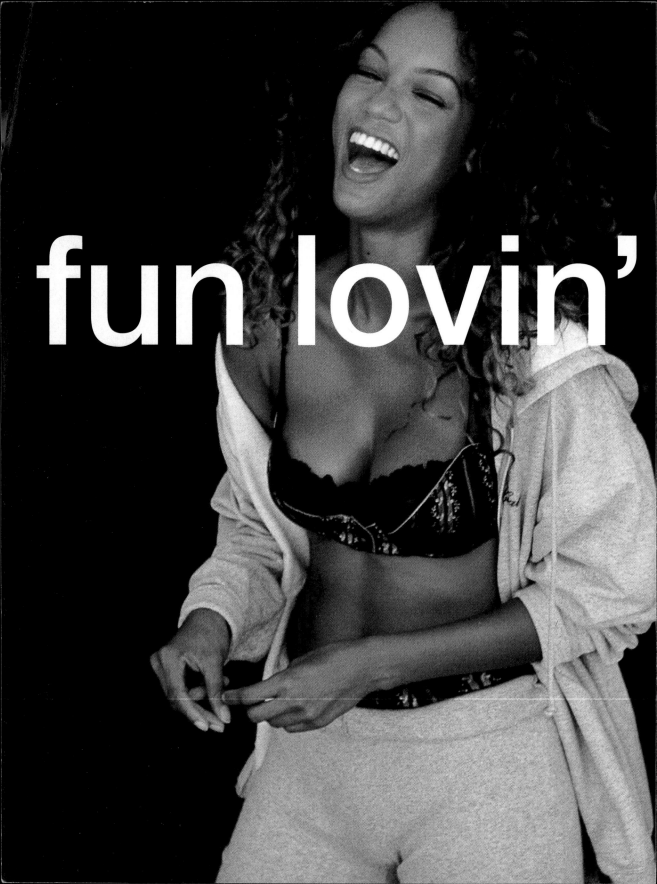